MW01489763

What My Patients Taught Me

A PHYSICIAN'S JOURNEY

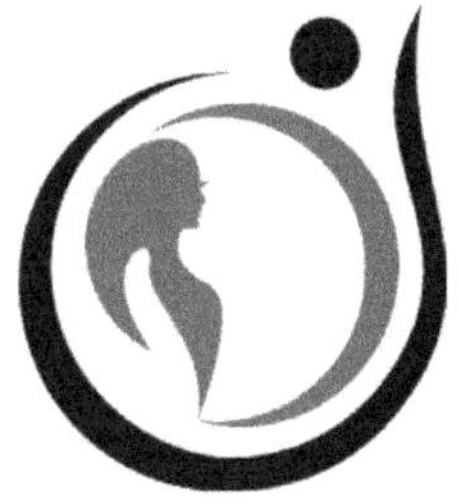

Lakshmi Gavini, M. D.

Obstetrician and Gynecologist

Dedicated to

All my patients

For showing me that every patient has a story, and behind every story, there is a person not defined by the diagnosis. For teaching me how to cherish the joys and face the challenges with the dignity of love, strength, hope, and faith.

My husband

Vinay Gavini for his love, support, and understanding, and for putting up with my long hours and many absent nights.

The memory of my parents

Mr. P.V.C Rao and Mrs. Krupavathi, for their love, guidance, and inspiration, and for instilling the belief in me that I could achieve anything, even having been born as a girl.

My family and friends who became family

For sustaining me during challenging times and for giving me the comfort of knowing that I could count on them.

V L Gavini Publishing LLC, MI

Printing and Distribution-Ingram Sparks

Book Cover Designed by Eric Keller

Lakshmi Gavini MD

What My Patients Taught Me-A Physician's Journey

ISBN 978-1-7321167-0-2

Lakshmi Gavini MD

URL: WWW.What My Patients Taught Me.com

E-Mail: Lakshmi Gavini@ What My Patients
Taught Me.Com

Library Of Congress

Control Number 2018904956

Disclaimer

To honor the privacy of all my patients, I used random initials for all patient stories. I wrote this book as a tribute to my patients.

Table of Contents

Introduction

At the end of the 51st year of my professional career in medicine and the 38th year of my clinical practice as an OB-GYN, I decided to retire. It was a very emotional time for me. As I was thinking about how to navigate this new, unfamiliar chapter in my life, I was pleasantly surprised and ultimately inspired, when some of my patients encouraged me to write a book.

As I wandered back into the past, reminiscing, I realized I had served not only as a witness to the significant changes in women's health over the past forty years but in the late 1970's and 80's, I had taken part in leading the revolutionary changes in obstetrical care. This professional journey started with the emotional requests of my patients, who—and rightfully so—wanted to have control over their childbirth experience.

They were disillusioned with the routine practices of the cold, sterile childbirth experience provided by the hospital and were looking for a nurturing bonding experience. This request for change propelled me onto the unexpected path of becoming one of the advocates for and an early practitioner of new childbirth practices at my hospital.

Looking back, I felt compelled to document how my patients' requests for change became my guiding light in adopting the practice of patient-centered care. While I was listening to them, I was learning from them, and this education continued for the remainder of my professional life (even when I disagreed in some situations).

This book is about my patients, whose stories made me think beyond what I had learned in medical school and residency training, an education which is, mostly, focused on medical diagnosis and treatment. As I understood my inadequacies and limitations as a physician, I learned that patients comprehend if physicians do not have all the answers.

My patients taught me how to recognize that there is a whole person behind every condition and each patient has a story. These life stories play a significant role in a patient's complicated decision-making process, a process that needs to be understood, and heard. Despite this understanding and to my disappointment, there were occasions where I failed to understand and validate my patients' concerns and needs.

As I was contemplating writing this book, I struggled with which stories to tell. I chose stories of patients whom I had followed for most of their lives. These were the stories that involved some of the more complex life-altering conditions, such as losing a baby, confronting a diagnosis of cancer, understanding the elusive science of depression, making difficult decisions before undergoing surgery, or merely trying to make sense of the changes during different stages of transition in life.

When faced with the challenges of illness, grief, or death, many people learn more about themselves. I was in awe of many of these women, who in the face of adversity were able to show grace under pressure, determination to heal with the strength of steel, and exhibit hope even when the odds were stacked against them.

During the recount of patient's life stories, I was inevitably led to narrate the contemporary history of medical and technological advances made in the specialty of OB-GYN over 40 years and my role in the early participation of those advances at my institution.

I address how the lessons I learned from my patients also helped me understand: the deficiencies in our healthcare system, the physician-patient disconnect, and the need for teamwork from all sides, while always placing the patient at the center of the hub. My desire to change and meet these challenges in our healthcare system led to my greater involvement in Ascension Health, one of the largest health systems in the country.

As I started to write this book, I was drawn to describe my journey growing up in India and my adopted home, the United States. In recounting this journey, I was surprised to learn how my life's experiences intertwined with my patients' experiences as I faced the challenges of my mother's illness, my father's dementia, cancer in the family, and my health issues.

My patients may never understand how they touched my life and how they inspired me to strive to become a better physician and hopefully a better person. It has been my honor to be a part of our journey together, and this book is my tribute to them from the depths of my heart.

Growing Up

Our parents deserve our honor and respect for giving us life itself. Beyond this, they almost always made countless sacrifices as they cared for and nurtured us through our infancy and childhood, provided us with the necessities of life, and nursed us through physical illness and the emotional stresses of growing up.

-- Ezra Taft Benson

I was born in a small town in India, with a population of 5,000. Born to two extraordinary middle-class parents, I am one of the three sisters and have no brothers. Our parents never made us feel less for being girls. In fact, they encouraged us to be independent and strong and gave us the confidence to do anything to which we set our minds. Our town had one high school, one hospital with a primary-care physician, one courthouse, and a police department. When I was growing up, most villages in India did not have a middle or high school or a physician. Our town served as the hub for high school education and healthcare for all the surrounding villages. Growing up under these conditions, we felt we were privileged.

Neither of my parents had finished high school, but I never regarded them as uneducated because they were very well read, engaged in politics, and were very knowledgeable about all the contemporary issues that affected our local community. My parents were not perfect, but we learned lessons from their exemplary way of living and the way they raised us. My father was a farmer and also worked as a contractor of infrastructure projects like roads, bridges, and buildings.

I was born just a few years after India's independence (1947); a lot was going on in rural India in my youth. My father was one of the most honest men that I ever knew. His construction projects were of the best quality, and the engineers loved his work. Interestingly, all the bids were in English; the system had not changed after India had gained independence from the British rule. He had figured out how to bid for the projects without any ability to read English. When I was in eighth grade, my father used to ask me to read the project proposals. I had no clue what I was reading, but he understood every word. As we were growing up, he subscribed to the English newspapers both to encourage us to read the news and to help us learn English. He had many friends who were professionals: engineers and physicians, lawyers, judges and police officers, and he was a person of influence in our community. My father was a community leader and was never too tired to help anybody. It did not matter to him whether a person was rich or poor. They might be coming to him for a big problem like a health or legal issue, because of his connections with physicians and lawyers at the district level, or for a small problem like a family squabble.

People came for his help at all hours; day or night, he was ready and willing to help.

Consequently, between his work and his involvement in community activities, we rarely saw our father while I was growing up. When he was home, many people wanted to talk to him and get his counsel, but most times, he was out of town taking care of the problems of others.

My mother was the center of our universe. My mother took care of us and everything else that needed taking care of in our home. Ours was a hectic household with cousins, aunts, and uncles visiting us frequently. My maternal grandmother often lived with us, too. My mother was very soft-spoken and never raised her voice, yet she was firm. I did not want to disappoint my mother or see her upset. She was very spiritual and had an unwavering faith in God. I never saw her cry, even during the most challenging times. I am very different from my mother in this regard; I am emotional and cry at the drop of a hat.

While my father was there for all the critical decisions in our lives, giving us his full support, my mother was the intellectual. She loved reading. She read many historical books and the ancient Hindu scriptures. When we were growing up, her primary focus was on us, and our education. My parents were different; unlike most parents in India, they did not find their daughters a burden, and made a conscious decision to educate us in spite of the significant criticism they received from our grandparents and other relatives. My parents were steadfast in following their plans and ignored everyone who disagreed. When I was young, I used to hear my mother telling her friends of my parents' plans to send me to medical school. I have no idea why they picked me, their middle child to be the doctor. I am sure this was not just my mother's idea; she would not have decided this without my father's support.

In India, despite all the advances made in the last 50 years, most parents think, even today, it is a burden to have girls because of the additional financial responsibilities that include marriage and negotiating dowry. During my youth, the girls growing up in India were required to behave in specific ways. Girls in India were not supposed to ride bikes or swim, nor were they supposed to play with or talk to boys. I was the quieter one of the sisters, but strong in both my ideas and my actions. I learned to ride a bike by myself, sometimes with the support of a young boy, who served as household help.

My parents were not aware of this new talent of mine until one day when my father saw me on the bike. I was worried and scared that he would reprimand me for my unacceptable behavior. Not only did my father not reproach me, but he was also very supportive when I got into accidents, causing minor scrapes to the others. He gave my victims money to get appropriate care. However, swimming was another matter entirely. I almost drowned when I tried to learn to swim in a freshwater pond, close to my house. I tried swimming classes after I came to the States, but I was never able to swim due to my fear of drowning, so I gave up on that idea.

During my school years, I was the youngest in my class, through the middle and high school years. I started 6th grade at the age of seven. In high school, we had an excellent headmaster, a follower of Mahatma Gandhi, who was part of the passive resistance freedom movement for India from the British rule. Mahatma Gandhi taught against any discrimination based on religion, caste, gender or economic standing. My headmaster followed the ideals and teachings of Mahatma Gandhi, even to the extent of marrying a widow, which was very unusual in Indian culture.

Most of our teachers were from the local area, and very average in their abilities to teach and motivate the students. Consequently, over 90% of the students from my class did not go on to college. When I was in high school, I loved math, may be influenced by my favorite math teacher, so I thought it might be interesting to be an engineer. My mother, in her wisdom, said that the engineering indeed belongs to a man's world and convinced me how hard it would be for me to survive in it. Subsequently, I decided to take biological sciences in college so that I could go to medical school, and I am so glad that I followed my mother's advice. I love medicine and have had no regrets.

In the 1960's there were no women engineers in India. Now it is widespread for girls to grow up and become engineers. I am not sure when that trend changed, but I am glad it did, so women have more choices. I think parental guidance is essential and helps children to move forward in the right direction as it helped me. Today, I see many high school graduates spending much money to go to college, who end up getting degrees that provide very little in the way of opportunity and result in much debt. I am not saying one should go into a field that one dislikes, but I do feel looking at different options and making wise choices, with the parental support, helps.

I had much fun growing up, surrounded by family and friends, and parents who loved three of us deeply. My father was a man who, in general, cared deeply but talked loudly and was easily angered When we were young children, however, he never spoke aloud to us girls.

My parents had planned for all three of us to go on to higher education. My older sister was the most social of the three of us. Despite my parents trying very hard to help her to get into college, she had no interest in going. Ultimately, both my parents accepted her decision, and she moved on. During her stay at home, before her marriage, they gave her the responsibilities of keeping an account of all the household finances, and she was given a monthly allowance for doing this accounting. She was encouraged by my parents to go to the post office to pay money order for the monthly subscription for the books. In those days in India, especially in villages, it was very uncommon for the girls to have the freedom to go beyond the confines of the home to take care of any chores. As a result of her experiences, she developed self-confidence and had all the tools she needed to be independent after she got married. My parents wanted her to be ready for the outside world, just like her two college-educated sisters. Today, she is married and has two sons, one of whom became a physician and the other, an engineer. My sister encouraged her children to aim for higher education, the same way my parents had urged us.

My younger sister, who is two years younger than me, is the most outgoing. She possesses a good sense of humor and leadership qualities. Everyone always adored her, and she is the life of every party, even now. When we were in school, our high school president and the several other class leaders were all boys. My headmaster, who was very progressive, decided that we should have a female leader for all the girls. He made my younger sister the first leader representing girls in our school.

She was a real leader and raised funds from the students to help a needy family who had lost their house in a fire. I was the naysayer about the fund-raising because I did not think the students would be able to give money to the cause. However, my father and our headmaster encouraged her to do it. She raised significant funds from the students, and we were all so proud of her leadership skills. My father helped with the rest, to build a home for that unfortunate family. My father was proud of her for what she had accomplished at such a young age.

My younger sister went to college and completed her graduate degree in political science. While teaching college, she fought at the state level, for the rights of all pregnant women, including a maternity leave of absence and job security, after she found out that she had no guarantee that her job would be safe during her maternity leave. She was able to get a temporary order in her favor. She is married to a man who fell in love with her during their high school years. She quit her job after ten years and chose to be a wife and mother. She has two beautiful daughters, one a physician and the other, an engineer.

Like any sisters, the three of us loved each other immensely, and, like many sisters, have sometimes disagreed about silly things that we did not remember for long. We have always come together to support each other in need. My two sisters remained in India, while I have been in the United States since December of 1972. The three of us are very close to this day, in spite of the physical distance between us. I have lived almost two-thirds of my life in the USA, which, not surprisingly, has created some cultural differences. However, in spite of these differences, we remain bound by the universal values we shared under my parents' guidance as we grew up. I talk to my sisters once a week. Even though we are 10,000 miles apart, we share our collective experiences with each other.

Many people influence a young person during his or her lifetime. For me, one of them was my headmaster; the other one was a local congressman. Our local congressman was a close family friend who was passionate and honest, a man who wanted to do what was right for his constituents. He never surrendered to corruption, despite the significant temptation around him. It was highly unusual to find a politician who did not succumb to corruption in India, so I admired his commitment to serve the people who had elected him most honestly. It is easy to say that is the way it should be, but in the real world that was not the way it was, especially not in India.

As I look back, it is easy for me to see that I had a great childhood, one not rich in wealth, but rich in sound values. My parents had friends from different faiths and religions. We belonged to the forward caste of Hindus, but we never looked at the caste or religion of our friends. As well as Hindu friends, we had Muslim and Christian friends. I am not sure the majority of the kids who grew up in India had such rich experiences. Growing up surrounded by mentors like my parents, my headmaster, and our congressman had more impact on me than I realized as a child.

Children are the product of their environment, good or bad. My family did not live in a utopian society. Many people were selfish or corrupt and did not share the same values as my parents, headmaster, congressman, and some of my teachers and community leaders. We were lucky to be surrounded by these human beings, who cared for the others and showed us the way. My father, unbeknownst to us, helped many poor students to go to school. We only found this out many years later, after his death. We were a middle-class family, but my parents did not hesitate to help others in their time of need.

My mother would take care of the needs at home, and my father took care of all external matters. The absence of my father during our childhood had an impact on me. I hated when my mother waited for my father to be home, not knowing what time and which day he would return. There was no efficient way of communicating with each other, long distance. Phone calls were onerous, and it was impractical to make them. I knew she would lie awake on the bed until he was home.

My mother, with all her reading of history and scriptures, admired many women leaders. While she was very traditional in fulfilling her roles as wife and mother, I think my mother was a "women's libber" in the best sense of the word, and understood the importance of education. She wanted her daughters to have the opportunity to excel and to enjoy the power and freedom that came with it. My mother loved our first female prime minister, Mrs. Indira Gandhi, and I was so happy when I took her to Delhi to visit Indira Gandhi and Mahatma Gandhi's memorials. It is hard to forget my travels with my mother to visit Taj Mahal in 1998. By that time, she was not in good health, but on the way, she gave me a history lesson about the Mughal rule in India. Mughal ruled India before the British, who ruled us until we achieved independence in 1947. I was embarrassed about my lack of knowledge of Indian history, while at the same time, I was delighted listening to my mother teach me, taking me back to being a young child looking to my mother, in awe of her grasp of history.

No other parents in our family were like our parents, and, as a result, all my cousins loved to visit our home. I can proudly say that I am still in awe of my parents; they were very much a part of the newly independent India with high hopes for their children and the country those children would inherit.

The Threat of Losing Mother: A Child's Perspective

During my childhood, one incident that had a profound impact on me was my mother's life-threatening illness. I want to share my experience, especially concerning the effects of the illness of a parent on a child's emotional health and the confusion it creates in the child's mind. When I was eight years old, my mother became very ill. The first couple of days of her illness, we children, did not realize how sick she was and how close she was to dying. After a couple of days, we noticed that many relatives had started showing up including aunts, uncles and our grandmother. There was a lot of talking, confusion, and sadness. I had never seen my father sad until that day when my mother was most critically ill.

I learned later that the local physician had informed my father that my mother might not make it. I can still see all our relatives looking grim and talking amongst themselves. I remember one of my relatives asking my father how he planned to take care of the three young children on his own. I was sad, confused, and scared as a young child with all that commotion going on around me. My older sister has since told me she felt the same way. My younger sister does not remember much about the event. Nobody thought to explain what was going on with us or to reassure us during this time of crisis. It is understandable that they did not think about our state of mind because my father and relatives were trying to deal with their fear and grief.

Finally, my father, with the support of our family, decided to take my mother to an American hospital, 50 kilometers from my town, managed by missionaries with an American physician on staff. I remember we traveled in a large van with my mother lying in a small bed and my father accompanied by three of us as well as other relatives. It was late evening by the time my father decided to take her to the American hospital, and the extra time it took to rent a van. It was monsoon season in India, and it was a rainy night. In the late 1950's, traveling 50 kilometers would have taken a minimum of five hours.

I am not sure how long it took us to reach the destination. I am sure we slept on the way. We woke up upon arriving at the hospital in the wee hours of the morning. Next thing I remember, my mother was taken away on a stretcher to be admitted to the hospital. I was talking to my older sister recently about this, and she told me that the staff thought we were delivering a person who had already died. Thank God, my mother did not die. I remember us peeking through the window while they were trying to insert an IV needle into my mother's dehydrated hand. After multiple attempts, they were able to start an IV.

The physician was a Caucasian woman, older in age. Of course, everyone looks older from a child's perspective. My memory was that the physician had grey hair, but now that I think about it, her hair could have been blond. Perhaps she was not so old, but I do remember that she possessed quite a calm, kind demeanor. My sisters and I did not understand what she was saying, but we were happy to see her taking care of our mother. All the nurses were very kind to our mother and us. My father rented a place for us to stay, which enabled us to visit our mother daily. Sometimes we even would sneak in to visit our mother more than once in a day, after visiting hours were over. The staff probably understood our need to see her and knew how lucky we were to have our mother survive an almost near-death experience.

After one week, when my mother was out of danger, my father decided to send my older sister and me back home with our grandmother, so we could go back to the school without missing too much time. We loved our grandmother, but that was the first time we had ever been at home without our mother. We felt sad that we could not see our mother and missed her very much but did not know how to talk about our feelings. It was a difficult time for us, not having our mother there to take care of all our physical and emotional needs. As children, we feel the safest with the daily routines of parental activities. It had nothing to do with my grandmother's care or a lack of love for us—she took great care of us, and we knew she loved us dearly—but the home did not feel like home, without our mother there.

It took one month for my mother to recover before she was discharged to come home. To this day, I am not sure what the diagnosis was; it most likely was some infection. We felt life was normal again with our mother walking through our home, talking to family members and friends, and guiding us like she always had. My grandmother stayed with us for an entire year to be of help to my mother. I am sure my grandmother felt better being "on site" to take care of her daughter who had escaped the fate of death. That is what mothers do, no matter how old the children become. My mother was the center of our universe, and once she was back, our universe was back to normal.

As I look back, I wonder what the best approach is to talk to children in time of a family or a community crisis. I think it would have been better if my father had reassuringly explained to us that while my mother was very sick, taking her to the hospital would make her better. In the 1950's, it would have been unheard of to have such a conversation, and even now, every parent handles it differently. Sometimes parents think that by not talking to their children, they are protecting them. However, parents do not realize that the children often have an innate ability to understand that something is wrong and are more afraid of the unknown than they would be in knowing the truth. Often, they are scared to ask questions and don't know what questions to ask. For, over the past 40 years, we have significantly improved our methods of identifying how to communicate with the children during a crisis with the help of psychologists.

A Story of Love: The Enigma of the Mother-Child Bond

Talking about my mother's illness reminded me of a patient during the early years of my practice. My partner and I had a patient eight months pregnant, who arrived at the hospital with a severe hemorrhage caused by placenta previa. Severe bleeding from placenta previa is a life-threatening condition for both the mother and the baby. We started a cesarean section to save both the mother's and baby's lives. During the procedure, despite having transfused multiple units of blood, the patient's blood pressure was very low, and we had to perform part of the surgery without anesthesia. After failing all the conservative treatments, we ultimately had to do a hysterectomy to control the uterine hemorrhage to save her life. We were relieved to see that both the mother and the baby survived the crisis.

The next day, during my visit with this patient in the ICU, she talked to me about her out-of-body experience and the white light she saw. She said she was looking at her own body from a corner of the room up close to the ceiling and could see everyone involved in her care working hard to revive her. Then she said, she saw her seven-year-old daughter and her husband begging her to come back. She believed that is what helped her to survive. In those days, we never heard of such white light and out-of-body experiences, which have been documented by many others since. I never could forget that encounter - the power of the mother's love for her child and the child's love for her mother that pulled the mother back and made her fight for her life.

I wonder if my mother experienced anything like it. I do not know if she did, but one thing I feel is that her love for us and our love for her brought her back from the shadow of death. I have observed over my years of practice, that so many outcomes go beyond any explanation of medical science. I have come to believe the crucial roles the mind and spirit play, roles that go beyond the body's physicality and the science that supports it.

A Story of Destiny

Thinking back now to my childhood, I know I was strongly inspired by American exceptionalism. At the time, I did not give much thought to how this exceptionalism had touched me in such a personal way. Colleges and hospitals run by the American religious organizations were the best in India. We were fortunate to have American physician volunteers who traveled far from the comfort of their own home, culture, and language to serve the people in need. In the 1960's, John F. Kennedy's Peace Corps program expanded the idea of helping others and took it to the next level of service with the education of the poor. After I came here, I had a few friends who said they had been part of the Peace Corps and what a great experience it was, how much they loved it, and how it made them better human beings. These peace corps friends inspired me, just as those American volunteers had many years ago in India.

I believe in these connections and call them "destiny." It is an interesting coincidence that an American physician volunteer saved my mother's life, and I came to America as a physician. This country, the United States of America, has given me so much, embracing me through my entire life. I love my adopted home, with all my heart, for all that it has given me.

College and Medical School

The capacity to learn is a gift; the ability to learn is a skill; the willingness to learn is a choice.

--- Brian Herbert

My college and medical school years were interesting. I had just become a teenager when I went to college for the next phase of my education before attending medical school. In college, students chose different courses. Depending on their grades and classes, students then can apply for admission into a medical, engineering or undergraduate college. My parents decided to enroll me in a Catholic all-girls college. Catholic schools, as well as Catholic hospitals, in my state of Andhra Pradesh, were known to be the best. My college was three hours away from home. Going to college was a significant adjustment and resulted in a considerable pressure to succeed for the students. There were many challenges for students moving from villages to adjust; a new place to live, a new school, new teachers and new classmates, and the difference in the medium of instruction from our native language to English.

My parents had concerns about these significant changes coming into my life at such an early age. They decided that it would be best for my mother and my sisters to move to my new college town. My parents made a great sacrifice during that one year in the life of our family. Though I did not realize at the time, it had to be very difficult for my mother, who was away from home, alone with no friends, and for my father, who was trying to manage his business responsibilities at home while making sure we were all doing well by visiting us frequently. I never heard them complain about it during that time or afterward. They wanted to make sure that their young daughter would not feel lost in this new environment without love and support. I was so fortunate to have such parents, who were not only thinking about my education but more importantly, cared about my physical and emotional well-being during the transformational years.

During my second year of college, my parents felt I was ready to live independently and had made the decision to move back home. I lived in the school dormitory. I had a few friends, who, had the same aspirations as I did, and we studied hard. Dormitory life gave me, as it provides many teenagers, the opportunity to grow up. Other than studying, we spent most of our time chatting and sharing in each other's lives like any teenagers would do. We managed to have a great time even in that restricted environment.

In my state of Andhra Pradesh, with a population, at that time, of 30 million people, there were six government and two private medical schools. Government schools were more highly rated and, accepted top students and the tuition fees were relatively insignificant. Most of the expenses were for the books, room, and board.

To get into medical school, one had to be in the top 90th percentile of one's college class. After I had completed my second year of college, I gained admission into Guntur Medical College, one of the best government-sponsored public medical schools in the state of Andhra Pradesh, located in southeastern part of India. I began medical school in 1965. Our class consisted of 150 students. Fifty percent of the students in our class were girls. It was good to know there were other parents, just like mine, who supported and encouraged their girls to go on to higher education.

The dichotomy in India is a stark contrast between the laws and the traditions. On the one hand, Indian society looked at girls as a burden while boys were given the highest importance in the family. On the other side, it is impressive to realize that, in 1965, 50 percent of my medical school class were girls, and that in 1966, India elected its first female prime minister, less than 20 years after India had gained independence in 1947. Life in India is very complicated and difficult to define, with such diversity of culture, caste, religion, regions, language, and wealth. It is much harder to describe women's roles and opportunities in India, the largest democracy in the world. Indian laws and the Indian government were always supportive and inclusive of all its citizens, including women. It is, and was, against the law to receive a dowry or to commit bigamy. Laws encouraged higher education for girls as well as minorities and were the part of a quota system for higher education.

However, the traditions and the culture were what held the country back. Many people did not follow the laws, and the enforcement of those laws was equally bad. In the last 40 years, there has been a significant increase in the middle class in India. In spite of these positive changes, some regions and most cultures in India keep girls and women in the background. So, in effect, this half, the female half, of the population has an insignificant role in making decisions for themselves or their families.

I started medical school in my mid-teens and was treated like an adult, and with some reverence. As I had in pre-medical school, I lived in a dormitory. It was not too hard to adjust because I had experienced dorm life the year before. During my medical school years; I am sorry to say I did not study hard. I focused more on having fun with my friends and less on studying. During those developmental years, I also thought more and more about the women's role in society, the unfair customs of the dowry system for girls, and discrimination based on caste, religion, and economic class. I started reading books that questioned society's ills. I transformed from being a young teenager to a young woman during my six and half years of medical education.

I know I challenged my parents significantly after I went to medical college. On some occasions, my father and I did not see eye to eye on many contemporary issues affecting the girls. When we were in serious disagreement, my mother always stepped in as the peacemaker. On the other hand, my mother and I used to talk about many contemporary issues, which held women in the background including love, marriage, caste, religion, politics, and dowry practices. We agreed on some and agreed to disagree on the others. As a teenager, I questioned everything, and she would explain and help me to understand the issues. I knew she was always there for my sisters and me. My mother was my close confidante, friend, and teacher. She guided me when I needed it and always gave me a quiet nod when I was on the right track.

During these medical school years, I became more spiritual but less religious, a person, with a firm belief in the Almighty but critical of the hypocrisy of the leadership of all organized religions. I did and still do have the highest respect and admiration, for those who live through the most challenging time in their lives with absolute faith in God and without questioning why. They are the real believers. My mother was one of them.

Medical education in India was different than in the United States. Being in the good graces of our professors was as crucial as doing well academically. A professor had significant control over a student's fate. Students were tested, one and a half years after studying anatomy, physiology, and biochemistry. If I failed, I could not start the next year until I passed the tests, given only every six months. So, this was a very critical time. I had not taken studying too seriously, and by the time summer came along, I knew I was in trouble. I stayed at school to study through the summer. It was scorching hot, and I had to eat at the restaurants because the dormitory cafeteria was closed for the summer. I do not know how I survived. Luckily there was another student who had stayed to study, so at least I had company. When the exams were all over, I had managed to pass all the tests that year.

After completing the basic medical science courses, we started our three clinical years. The clinical years were how a student got to try on the feeling of being a "doctor." In the morning, we were scheduled to examine patients and participate in an educational session led by the postgraduate students or assistant professors and attended the classroom lectures in the afternoon. We had great professors, who were highly qualified. Most of them were fellows of the Royal College of Medicine, Surgery, OB-GYN, and Pediatrics and had passed fellowship exams in England. Most female professors were in OB-GYN although some had chosen pediatrics. Very few men specialized in OB-GYN. During these three years, besides learning the basics of general medicine, general surgery, OB-GYN, and Pediatrics, we were also taught pharmacology and pathology. Pharmacology taught us about the function of different drugs and how the drugs help in the treatment of medical conditions. Pathology was the study of diseases and how they caused the abnormal functioning of different systems in the human body.

During clinical rotations in the hospital, as students, we were expected to see one patient assigned to us for that day. Groups of students were assigned to the unit, to take the history, to do a physical exam and to present the case to a postgraduate student, who was the equivalent to a resident physician in the U.S. or an assistant professor. All our discussions about the case were at the bedside, and we, the students, presented the patient's symptoms and our physical examination findings, followed by the lengthy discussions about diagnosis and treatment, without acknowledging the patient once. I do not remember at any time during these clinical rounds, that we, the students, looked at the suffering human being as a person or gave a thought about his or her fears and feelings or his or her background. A doctor's response was to diagnose and treat the illness without any explanation of the treatment plan to the patient. The patient was just a bystander, while we were making life-and-death treatment decisions for him/her. Most of the patients were poor and uneducated, and one could argue the practical difficulties of explaining a complex condition or treatment to this population. Kind words could have gone a long way to providing comfort to the patients, but teaching the humanity in medicine was not part of the curriculum then.

If the outcomes were poor, patients and families accepted it as fate, without any questions. It was the lack of empathy that I remember the most. One day during morning rounds, a nurse reported that one of our patients who had delivered the night before died of postpartum hemorrhage. Surprisingly, nobody blinked an eye, and all of us moved on to discuss the next patient. This incident reminded me of an event before I was born when my mother almost lost her life from postpartum hemorrhage during the birth of what would have been the only son of my parents. The baby boy did not survive the birth. My mother only survived because of the excellent care provided by a local physician. I felt terrible about the loss of that other mother, our patient, who had died from the postpartum hemorrhage.

We never saw the family of that mother. Usually, it was the family members who supported each other, during such a time of crisis, without a word of comfort from the physicians. That is how we learned; the doctors were responsible for diagnosing and treating, hoping for good outcomes. We were not taught the tools to think beyond the disease or condition we were addressing. This same cycle of learning continues today. How a physician communicates with a patient is learned by observation, allowing for only very subtle changes between one generation of physicians to the next.

I did complete my medical school on time, without failing any exams, in spite of my shortcomings as a serious student of medicine. After medical school, to get our medical degree, we each were required to work as a house surgeon in the hospital for one year. House Surgeon is the equivalent to a rotating internship in the U.S., with the mandatory rotations of internal medicine, general surgery, ob-gyn, pediatrics and some electives. Our primary responsibility was to see all the patients in the unit, accompanying the post-graduate students assigned to that unit, making notes of the patient's condition and determining a treatment plan. Later in the day, assistant professors made rounds with the post-graduates and house surgeons to make sure the diagnosis and treatment plan was acceptable. Few times a week, a professor also made bedside rounds. House surgeons were also responsible for executing the orders, doing some basic bedside labs, drawing the blood and, most often, giving the injections.

I loved the idea of bedside rounds. Most of the diagnoses were made, purely by considering the patient's history and a clinical exam. Our professor's ability to accurately make a clinical diagnosis by looking at the patient was phenomenal. We used to have "spot diagnosis" challenges. These bedside rounds were most helpful in treating the patients, as the physician team was all on the same page regarding the diagnosis and in executing the treatment plan.

I also observed how the whole system worked following the hierarchy. No one could question the decisions of a physician who held a superior position. In spite of the professors' sarcasm or condescending manner, directed primarily toward their post-graduate students and assistant professors, we learned a great deal from them.

"Death & Dying 101" Has a Face

As house surgeons, we saw many patients who were dying from all kinds of different diseases. Among these dying patients were many young children who were suffering from dehydration, malnutrition, and especially, meningitis. In spite of our best efforts in treating these children, they were already in the terminal phase of the disease when their parents brought them to the hospital, and some children died. We felt sad to see the parents' agony but accepted the outcomes because there was nothing more we could do. We did not know then about the stages of grief, and it was not part of the curriculum to address how to talk to grieving parents. There was no curriculum describing the stages of grief, until Elisabeth Kübler-Ross described them in her book *On Death and Dying: What the Dying*

Have to Teach Doctors, Nurses, Clergy and Their Own Families in 1969 (Scribner).

During my house surgeon year, one patient had a significant impact on me. While I was doing my internal - medicine rotation, a young man was admitted to the hospital for severe fatigue, and we diagnosed him with aplastic anemia, a form of blood cancer. This form of cancer prevents the patient's bone marrow from producing the red blood cells, the white blood cells, and the platelets, which are vital for carrying oxygen, for preventing infections and abnormal bleeding. In those days, there was no treatment for this type of cancer except to give blood transfusions. The patient was a Ph.D. student in pharmacology, and he was working with the chemicals that were implicated in his cancer. We all knew he was going to die. I am not sure if any of the senior physicians ever explained his diagnosis or prognosis to him. I saw him daily for 30 days during my rotation and followed his declining condition. I remember him being very nice and humble. He never complained or questioned his treatment and, in fact, accepted our treatment with grace.

After 30 days, I changed to a different unit. I went back to see the patient with aplastic anemia regularly until the patient died a month later. By the time he died, he had become blind and appeared unaware of his surroundings. I wondered what he had known about his condition. He was highly educated, and, at some level, he had to know about his prognosis. It was possible, he had hoped for a miracle against all the odds, and that hope had triumphed over his fear. Why do I remember him more than others who lost their life? Was it because he was young—in his mid-20s'—and educated? Was it because of his calm demeanor in the face of his grave diagnosis? Alternatively, could it be because his future was cut short by the very research he was doing to find new drugs to cure diseases?

Years later, I lost my cousin to acute leukemia at age 40. He was treated, at the MD Anderson Cancer Center in Houston. My cousin reminded me again of my patient of over 40 years earlier, who had lost his life to a similar form of blood cancer. I wondered why my cousin's treatment did not work, while others receiving the same treatment survived the same disease. In spite of all the scientific advances we have made in medicine, we have still not conquered an understanding of the nuances of the individual genetic makeup of cancer and the resulting different responses to the same treatment of the same disease. These two young men taught me more about human spirit than they did about their conditions.

Weighing Choices, Making Decisions

On a personal front, my house surgeon year was my most important one, and it changed the path of my future. At the end of six and half years, after the completion of the house surgeon, we finally received our medical degrees. My classmates chose different paths. Some went on to practice as primary care physicians. Most, however, either decided to go for post-graduate education in one of their favorite specialties or chose to take the exam to make them eligible to do specialty training in the U.S. My best friend, who was two years ahead of me Ramana, had already gone to U.S.A for further education.

I never wanted to be too far from my family, especially my mother, so I decided to stay in India and planned to go into a post-graduation program. My parents were thrilled with this plan, and I stayed at home with my parents for about four months, before starting the post-graduate education. During this time at home, I worked with one of the local doctors, helping him see patients. My parents were happy to see me helping friends and families in the area. It was a small town, and word spread fast. They were very proud parents of a physician daughter and enjoyed hearing the praise and feedback from their friends. Though it was a short-term plan until my admission into the post-graduation program, my parents were enjoying my time at home with them. Like most other young people, as much as I loved my mother, I could not wait to go back to school to be with my friends. During the process of applying for post-graduation, I toyed with the idea of going into general surgery.

When I was a house surgeon, I had loved the surgery rotation. I was thinking aloud one evening while sitting with my mother about the possible option of going into general surgery for post-graduation. You have to understand; I had never seen a female professor in general surgery. Women physicians primarily chose OB-GYN or pediatrics, with a few of them going into internal medicine. In fact, my sister-in-law was one of the first women to go into internal medicine in our university. My mother asked me one question: If I were to go into general surgery, would patients accept me, as a woman, as a surgeon, and if they did not, how would that make me feel? In a very subtle way, my mother was thinking aloud about the acceptance of a woman as a surgeon in the society for what is considered as a man's field. So, I decided to apply to the OB-GYN program.

During this same year, my older sister got married into a traditional, arranged marriage. I accepted my sister's wedding, understanding her limited options, given that she lived at home. It was time for me to get married. During my medical school years, I had gotten some proposals for marriage, but I had a definite opinion about love and marriage. I had to know and love my future husband, and he would need to share my values and be willing to accept no dowry.

We did not have too many young men who would not ask for and expect a dowry. Male doctors received a large dowry. Wealthy fathers loved providing a large dowry to physicians who would bring status to the family and high financial security to their daughters. Most physicians made good money and were considered affluent in the community. A wife's dowry was often used as seed money to start her husband's medical practice. Most medical students came from a middle-class background and did not have the financial means to start a medical practice on their own. The dowry could also be used to help other members of the family if the young man came from a background of limited financial means. Very few men, when I was of marriageable age, would have gone along with the idea of receiving no dowry.

Changing Course

When I was a house surgeon, I had met my husband-to-be, Vinay entirely by accident. His sister was the assistant professor of internal medicine at my school, but I had never worked with her. One of my husband's cousins was a classmate of mine, and while I had heard of him from this cousin of his, I had never met him. My future husband knew nothing about me. We went to different medical schools, but his family lived in the same city where I went to medical school.

I met Vinay on a train. I was planning to travel to attend the wedding of one of my classmates and a friend since pre-medical school years. Vinay, who knew the groom, was planning to attend the same wedding. I had been lazy about making reservations for a sleeping berth to accommodate the all-night trip. His cousin informed me that Vinay had one extra ticket, and if I wanted it, Vinay could give me the ticket at the railway station. I met Vinay on the railway station platform at a mutually agreed spot. Railway stations in India are like a scene much like that of a carnival. It usually was continually bustling with the sounds of arriving and departing trains, noisy overhead announcements, and even louder sales pitches from vendors who had set up to capture the travelers' attention, and, of course, lots and lots of people, jostling each other and sometimes running to catch their trains. What I first noticed when I met Vinay were his good looks and friendly smile. We introduced ourselves to each other, he gave me a ticket, and I gave him the money that I owed him. Then, we boarded the train together.

We ended up in the same compartment, and we talked all night. We talked about our schools, our professors, and our friends. There was a lot to talk about, being from different medical schools. I found him fascinating, and I enjoyed his company. The next morning, we attended the wedding, and as we were leaving, Vinay asked me if I would mind if he wrote letters to me. I was happy to know that he wanted to continue the friendship and said I would like that.

Starting our relationship off with letters was a great way to get to know each other. We exchanged ideas about different issues in society and our beliefs. He was different from any of the other young men I knew. He was the only one who played guitar, liked pop music, and talked about the Beatles, Harry Belafonte, and other musicians. That got my attention. I did not know much about the guitar, the music, the musicians, but I found him very interesting.

Friendship led to courtship. I loved the way he cared about his family. He came from a large family with seven children, including two very young sisters. His family was a middle-class family like ours, but his parents were older than mine. His older sister was already in the U.S., taking on some of the family's responsibilities.

We both talked about our families extensively. He wanted to make sure that I would be up to taking on the responsibility of his younger sisters. He was so honest with me in discussing his family matters, and I loved him even more for his commitment to his family. I knew I could always depend on him, and I said yes to his proposal. At that time, my parents did not even know that I was dating him. They had only met him once when I invited him to attend my sister's wedding.

During this initial year of friendship with Vinay, I had already enrolled in a post-graduation course in obstetrics and gynecology. During our conversations, Vinay expressed keen interest in exploring different cultures and explicitly said he wanted to go to the U.S.A for further education. After much discussion, I agreed to go along with Vinay's plan. The time had come to announce this plan to my parents. I wrote a letter to my parents about my decision to get married and told them about my fiancé and our plans to go to the U.S.A. I also informed them of my plans to discontinue my post-graduate studies to get ready for the qualification exam in America. In that letter, I did say that I would not proceed without their blessings. Our plan to move to the U.S. was one time in my life I disappointed my parents. I believe I broke my parents' hearts when they learned of our plans. They had high hopes that after my post-graduation experience, I would return to my village and set up a practice to help people there. They were naturally upset that they would not be able to see their daughter for long periods of time. I was the only one in my generation, on either side of my family, to leave India for a new life.

My mother was also disappointed that I was discontinuing OB-GYN postgraduate course. I promised my mother that I would continue to study the OB-GYN specialty in the U.S., not being aware of how difficult it would be as a woman to get admission into OB-GYN.

In later years, when my parents visited me a few times, they were very proud of me and happy that I had done well. They came to understand how much I loved my life as well as the practice of medicine in the U.S. I do not think they ever stopped feeling the emptiness caused by my absence, and that was one thing I could not change. Now that I have gotten older and have lived a lifetime, I understand my parents' agony better, as a result of being so far away from me. The separation must have been especially hard for my mother, whose entire life revolved around her children.

My parents, however, had no objection to our marriage, and fortunately, Vinay's parents and the rest of his family did not have any issues to a daughter-in-law not bringing any dowry with her. So, we got married with the blessings from both sets of our parents and other family members.

After our marriage, I stayed with my in-laws for three months while we were preparing for the qualification exam. My father-in-law was an absolute gentleman, and while my mother-in-law was tough and independent, she was always kind to me.

During the three months spent in their home, I had much fun with my two younger sisters-in-law and grew very fond of them. My in-laws were very supportive of us going to the U.S. My father-in-law was a businessman who had traveled many countries before he lost his wealth in the business and settled down to be an insurance salesman to support his large family. He loved his children and encouraged them to travel abroad and take advantage of what the world has to offer.

About four months after we got married, with the support and encouragement of my older sister-in-law, in December of 1972, we arrived in the U.S.

Internship and Residency

Education is not the learning of facts,
but the training of the mind to think.
--Albert Einstein

In December 1972, after arriving in the U.S., the first thing on our minds was to study and prepare for the ECFMG (Educational Council for Foreign Medical Graduate) exam. After much preparation and long hours of studying, Vinay and I took and passed the exam in June 1973. We both were ecstatic that we had passed the exam and could start making plans for our future. Passing the ECFMG was a significant milestone for us to forge ahead with our plans. The next step in that process was to apply for internships. The process is the same to this day. NRMP (National Residency Matching Program) is an American-based non-governmental organization started in 1952 to help match the medical school graduates with the residency programs. Most of the national medical organizations sponsor NRMP. We decided to do a "couples match," which meant we would go to the hospital that was a match for both of us. Naturally, we wanted to live in the same city, and we were delighted to know that we were able to do that through the couples-matching program.

The process of matching a medical student to a hospital for an internship is very complicated. The student gains admission into the program when the student and the hospital list each other as a preferred choice. It took much of the 2nd half of June '73 and 1st half '74 for the matching process to complete before we could begin the post-graduate training as interns. Luckily, both of us succeeded in being matched to Mt. Carmel Mercy Hospital in Detroit. We were excited to start our new life together by working at the same hospital.

Learning about American Politics from Watergate Trial

My sister-in-law was working as an internist in a V.A. hospital in Clarksburg, West Virginia, and I stayed with her until we settled. I worked for few months filling temporary positions in the emergency room in West Virginia, and my husband went back to India to complete his rotating internship obligations in the medical program in India before we both started our internships in July of 1974. During that one-year gap, I had plenty of time on my hands with very little to do all day. In 1973, I spent most of my time watching TV. The Watergate investigation was in high gear, and I watched the broadcasting of the Watergate hearings.

When I was in India, I was always interested in the political process, but this was something different. I glued myself to the TV during the entire telecast of the Senate hearings, chaired by Senator Sam Erwin. The courage and honor that the senators displayed during those hearings were beyond anything I had heard or read, in India. Two young investigative reporters, Bob Woodward and Carl Bernstein, from the Washington Post, were allowed to report the possible involvement of most influential people in the government, with the support of Ben Bradlee, editor-in-chief, and Katherine Graham, publisher of the Washington Post. Katherine Graham was a phenomenally gutsy lady. Years later, when I read her autobiography, I understood why she was bold and gutsy and what she had to endure in her life. She is one of my heroes. In the end, the entire country witnessed the tragic outcome of seeing the president of the U.S., the most powerful political leader in the world, forced to resign from the office. In India, that would never have happened. During all my years growing up in India, no political leaders had been held responsible or forced to resign from their positions for illegal activities that, in many cases, were transgressions much worse than those involved in the Watergate debacle. I knew then that the U.S. was an extraordinary country. I fell in love with it then, and it is a love story that continues to this day.

Finally! Arriving in "The D"

We both moved to Detroit at the end of June 1974 to start our rotating internships. During the rotating internship, we were assigned to different specialties every couple of months; some were mandatory, and the others were electives. The goal of the internship was to understand the basic concepts of diagnosis and the treatment of the conditions affecting the different systems of the human being. There was an orientation program for two days led by two chief residents who oversaw all the interns and the residents. The orientation included orienting the interns to the hospital, night calls, beepers, lockers, and other such logistics.

Chief residents Dr. Abdulla and Dr. Canedo were excellent teachers and were very kind to the interns. They made sure married couples had night-duty calls on the same night shift. We were very grateful for that gesture of kindness. The system of learning medicine was so different in the U.S. when compared to the training in India. We were given significant responsibilities in the patient evaluation, and care including, taking the patient's history, performing the physical exam, and coming up with a treatment plan before discussing a final plan with the resident physician-in-training. In some routine cases, we could decide on a final plan independently. We learned quickly with this type of training. During the year of internship, we had to make plans for the residency specialty training for next year. In 1974, there was no matching program for residencies, so by September, we had to decide our specialty of choice and start the application process. Interns applied to many hospitals all over the country to have more options of getting into the specialty of their choice. Some medical specialties were harder than the others to get into, especially for foreign medical graduates, which was understandable. I wanted to specialize in OB-GYN, so during my internship, I chose an OB-GYN rotation as my first choice, so I would have a better chance of getting into an OB-GYN program.

Mt. Carmel Mercy Hospital had only gynecology service, no obstetrics. After completing my GYN rotation, I was asked to go to an affiliated institution, Providence Hospital in Southfield, for my OB rotation. Providence had a full-fledged OB-GYN residency program. I loved this rotation. My chief resident was Dr. Rick Wilson. They were all very helpful to me. At Providence Hospital, I mostly worked with Dr. Wilson, and at Mt. Carmel Mercy Hospital, I worked with Dr. Prayong. I could perform Dilation and Curettage (D&C) and be able to second-assist in hysterectomies. The OB-GYN program at Providence Hospital was phenomenal. As an intern, I was expected to assess patients in labor and assist in forceps deliveries. Labor and delivery nurses played a vital role in the preliminary assessment of patients, as they are now.

When I started my internship, I worked very hard, but I was shy and quiet. During my rotation in obstetrics, in spite of my shyness, nurses reached out to me and were very kind to me. They taught me so much and played a significant role in my understanding and assessment of laboring patients. As an intern, I worked with the other residents in labor and delivery and also evaluated the patients in the emergency room under resident supervision.

The Case that Made the Difference

In the emergency room, it was not unusual for patients to arrive at the hospital in shock with hemorrhaging inside, from a ruptured tubal pregnancy. If it goes undiagnosed, it was/and is a life-threatening condition. Now we have many early diagnostic tools to help to prevent rupture of a tubal pregnancy, but in 1974, there were no noninvasive diagnostic tools to employ before the fallopian tube ruptured. Many patients arrived at the emergency room in shock.

One time, I was the only intern on a night duty call with Dr. Rick Wilson, and he asked me to see a patient who came to the emergency room with severe abdominal pain. I was by myself when I assessed this patient. After the exam, I was sure she needed to have a test called culdocentesis to determine if she had a tubal pregnancy that had ruptured and was leaking blood into the abdomen or if she had a pelvic infection that had formed an abscess with pus. A ruptured tubal pregnancy requires surgery; whereas an abscess requires intravenous antibiotics. Culdocentesis is a painful procedure, for which I needed to insert a needle into the vagina, the space between the cervix and the rectum. I had informed the patient that the procedure was necessary, to determine the exact diagnosis. Almost all patients who undergo culdocentesis, scream with pain, as did this patient of mine. I aspirated pus and was very excited that I had made the accurate diagnosis. At that point, I was thinking less about the patient, and I was more excited about having made the diagnosis without any supervision. I showed very little empathy toward the patient, who was going through this painful procedure and who possibly harbored fears about this life-threatening diagnosis.

I called Dr. Rick Wilson to inform him of my diagnosis. He was impressed with my assessment and diagnosis, and,

I think, this incident might have helped me get into the OB-GYN residency program at Providence Hospital.

During my internship year, my priorities were learning patient care and practice methods that included assessment and diagnosis of different medical conditions. I did not focus on the cultural background or the emotional status of patients that we were treating. At that time, this was the typical attitude of an intern. We tended to focus on the patient's condition rather than the patient as a person. Moreover, it was more challenging to have an emotional connection with the patients, while also trying to learn a new culture. For the new doctors that came from different countries with various backgrounds and the customs, no orientation existed to introduce the American culture. Unfortunately, that is still true, even today. I believe it would be a great start to have a cultural orientation classes for foreign medical graduates of different cultures and teach them the importance of looking at the patient as a person, not merely as a condition, and helping them to learn how to approach and connect with their patients.

OB-GYN: A Man's Specialty

I liked OB-GYN from the very beginning of my internship year; besides, I had promised my mother that I would continue my postgraduate studies in OB-GYN. Vinay was very supportive and encouraged me to go into whatever specialty I wanted to. I knew how difficult it would be for me to get into an OB-GYN residency. In 1974, OB-GYN physicians were predominantly men. I was at a distinct disadvantage in several ways: in being a woman, a foreign medical graduate, and, at five feet tall, 90 pounds, and small in stature. The OB-GYN specialty was and still is a highly demanding field involving long hours and a high-stress environment.

However, in the mid- 70's, more women started choosing OB-GYN as a specialty. I applied during this transition time. I wanted to stay in Detroit. In fact, I only applied to Providence Hospital's OB-GYN residency program. If Providence Hospital did not accept me into its program, I would have had no other recourse and would have lost an entire year. To my advantage, I had applied for the residency program while I was still at Providence Hospital during my OB-GYN internship rotation. Waiting to hear if I gained admission was a very stressful time, both for me individually and for us as a couple. The chairman of the department was Dr. Donald Krohn, and the program director was Dr. Henry Maicki. Unfortunately, I had very little interaction with either one of them during my rotation at Providence Hospital.

Two weeks after I applied, I received a rejection letter from Providence Hospital's department of education. It is hard to express the disappointment and feeling of rejection, especially after most of the residents felt I was doing a good job. The next day, at work I talked to the residents, who advised me to speak to the chairman, Dr. Krohn. I mustered the courage to call the chairman's office and made an appointment to talk to him. My goal was to explain to him that I received a rejection letter from the Providence OB-GYN residency program and to plead with him for reconsideration. On the day of my appointment, I was worrying all day about what to say to him. Especially being shy, I was worried about my ability to express my passion for OB-GYN. During the meeting, to my surprise, he said that he had heard of my interest in OB-GYN residency from Dr. Wilson. He said that Dr. Wilson, as chief resident of the program, had advised him to consider me for the residency. I never even had the opportunity to explain to him about having already been rejected.

He, however, did express his reservation about whether I would have the stamina to meet the demands of this highly stressful and demanding field. He was also concerned about whether I would be able to perform forceps deliveries, being a petite woman. I reassured him that I could do forceps deliveries, and, in fact, I had done a few as an intern. He said he would give me a one-year contract and would reevaluate me at the end of the year, renewing my contract dependent on my performance. I was so excited about the opportunity he had given me; I did not worry about the offer being for only one year. I think he was genuinely concerned about whether I had the stamina to meet the demands of this specialty. He never called me in for reevaluation at the end of the first year. I am forever grateful to Dr. Donald Krohn and to the now-deceased Dr. Richard Wilson for their roles in helping me to realize my dream. I believe there are no coincidences and that things happen for a reason. It happened to be one of those things that changed the direction of my life forever.

Meanwhile, my husband went through rotations including anesthesia and pediatrics. He was not sure what specialty interested him. He knew he did not want to do internal medicine, general surgery, or radiology. With the encouragement and support of the chief of anesthesiology at Mt. Caramel Mercy Hospital, Dr. Holt, Vinay went for an interview for the anesthesiology residency at the University of Michigan and was accepted. After much consideration, he decided to go into pediatrics. Dr. Montgomery, chairman of the pediatrics residency at Mt. Carmel Mercy Hospital, offered him a position, and he accepted.

Finally, on July 1st, 1975, Vinay and I started our residency programs in our chosen fields. During the three years of my residency, I worked with many excellent attending physicians. They were great teachers and clinicians. As residents, we worked very closely with the program director, Dr. Henry Maicki. He became my mentor as well as my friend. Dr.Gene Otlewski, Dr.ConnieTubbs, and Dr.Jim Kornmessor were the other attending physicians who played a significant role in my career, who became my friends.

Obstetrics was and is still a highly demanding and stressful field. During the residency program, we learned from assisting attending physicians during deliveries and surgeries. Senior residents were responsible for the patient care on the unit and did most of the teaching to junior residents and medical students. Didactic sessions were held for about three hours a week. The rest was up to us, which amounted to a lot of self-learning and reading. The three years of residency were very intense.

Obstetricians must think about two patients: the mother and the baby. The health of the baby depends on the health of the placenta, which depends on the health of the mother. The placenta is the most vital organ, the interface connecting the mother and the baby. The placenta via the umbilical cord is responsible for the blood circulation of the baby, that is responsible for the nourishment, oxygenation, and growth of the baby. Multiple conditions can impact a mother's or baby 's health anytime during the nine months of pregnancy. There are occasions when physicians have to choose a mother's life over the baby's. Things can go wrong at any moment in the labor and delivery unit. It is indeed a miracle that most babies are born healthy.

To make sure that our care was consistent, we had to follow specified routines. We informed patients of what was the treatment plan and the procedure, but we never gave the patient an opportunity for input. The 1970s was the era of "Doctor-Knows-Best," and questions from patients were not encouraged. Once we determined that the patient was in labor, routinely her pubic hair was shaven, and she received a soapsuds enema to make sure her bowels were empty before the delivery. We believed that both practices reduced infection. We learned later that shaving increases the risk of infection and a soapsuds enema does not make any difference in keeping the delivery area clean.

Patients were given fluids intravenously to avoid dehydration. They were not allowed to eat or drink from the time of admission until after delivery, to prevent complications of food aspiration, in case if they needed anesthesia for an emergency. A patient had to lie on her back through the entire labor process unless she had to run to the bathroom *across the hall* when the soapsuds enema finally started working. These routine practices were accepted and supported by OB-GYN physicians across the country.

We did have great teachers, who taught us how to evaluate and treat emergencies during labor and delivery, apply forceps, perform cesarean sections, and do meticulous episiotomy repairs. We were held responsible and got unhappy comments from the attending physicians for any infractions of the routine processes.

During my training years, a husband was not allowed to be in the room with his laboring wife. Most of the husbands did not want to be in the labor room and were scared, felt helpless, and didn't know how to help their laboring wives with the pain. If any husband wanted to be in the room to support his wife, we thought he was weird, and he was asked to leave the room for every exam.

Nurses spent more time with patients for assessment of labor and monitored the baby at regular intervals. Residents made rounds every one to two hours or when needed to make sure that the labor was progressing appropriately and that the baby was not showing any signs of stress. Attending physicians came in only when the patient was ready for delivery or any critical events were affecting the mother or baby.

I cannot imagine now, how scared those mothers must have been with no support. Mothers were going through most of the labor all alone, with very little preparation for this significantly painful and life-altering event. When appropriate, patients received medication for pain. The first stage of labor is when the cervix dilated to ten centimeters. During the second stage of labor, the patient should push during the labor contractions to deliver the baby. Nurses were at the mother's bedside during the second stage to guide her on how to push the baby. It is hard work; no wonder we called it labor! When ready for delivery, we moved patients from the labor room to the delivery room, gave them spinal anesthesia, and the delivery process was completed using forceps after making an episiotomy (a cut made in the woman's perineum. The process I described was all routine delivery practice in the 1970s.

It was considered a failure on our part if the woman had a natural childbirth, and for not timing the administration of the spinal anesthesia. We administered spinal anesthesia for all vaginal deliveries. Spinal anesthesia helped to prevent the natural maternal urge to push the baby. It gave enough time for the attending physician to come in and complete the delivery with forceps after performing an episiotomy). I still hear the sounds of wheeling beds with the laboring woman grunting to push, while running through the hallways to the delivery room, as we loudly and repeatedly saying to the patients "Don't push, Don't push" so we could administer the spinal anesthesia. We were reprimanded by the attending physicians if a patient was unable to control the natural urge to push and ended up having the baby naturally. Believe it or not, we had to write up a report, to substantiate how a natural birth occurred before getting the spinal anesthesia.

For many centuries, the laboring woman was supported and nurtured by the other women and, was given words of comfort and support to help with the intensity of labor and birth. In labor and delivery, the most empowering moment of childbirth was turned entirely into a litany of procedures, routines, clinical diagnosis, and medical treatment. We had very little understanding of how to support or address the nurturing aspects of this most transformational emotional event in a couple's life.

Childbirth, from the beginning of times, was a life-or-death event for both mother and baby, and many babies and mothers did not survive it. It is true, having babies in the hospital saved many mothers' and babies' lives. However, some of the routines we used in the hospital did not make sense, like, after the delivery, we used to give the mother Valium, a medication for relaxation, and the baby was whisked away to a warmer and after a brief checkup was transferred to the nursery for 24 hours. The mother never got to see the baby after he/she was born and could not hold the baby for 24 hours. This policy was in place to prevent newborn infections. If any mother requested to keep the baby, she was considered to be a troublemaker. Most patients accepted this process and were respectful of the idea that doctors knew best. This most intense emotional nurturing experience that should have been a crowning joy by holding and loving the baby was lost entirely in this sterile and unemotional experience.

We worked in a highly demanding field, and we were expected to perform at the highest level to achieve the perfect outcome. There was no place for "failure,"whether it is big or small. Hospitals and physicians developed stringent policies and routine orders that were believed to ensure the safety of the mother and baby. Consequently, there was never a dull moment in the labor and delivery unit. We were running either to examine the woman in labor or to administer spinal anesthesia to assist a mother ready to deliver or to evaluate the fetal heart tones, who was suddenly showing signs of distress. Meanwhile, an emergency could happen any time with a patient wheeled in actively bleeding, or get a call to see a patient in the emergency room requiring immediate attention. We had to be ready to handle a crisis at any moment and learn to triage appropriately, providing gentle guidance to the rest of the team to ensure the best outcomes. I loved obstetrics.

Gynecology service was entirely different. In-patient gynecology services were for patients who would be undergoing gynecology surgeries as well as some patients who needed medical treatment in the hospital. All patients were admitted to the hospital the day before surgery. Residents evaluated the patients by taking their histories, doing physical exams, and ordering tests that were appropriate for the operation with the approval of the attending physicians. These evaluations helped us to get to know the patient and to, understand the diagnosis and the decision-making process that had led to the surgery.

During the past 30 years, with the improvement in the pre-operative processes, patients do not get admitted to the hospital the night before. Residents do not get to see the patient until an hour before surgery and, consequently, know very little about the patient. I am not suggesting we should go back in time. The current process is better for the patients, but the residents do not have time to understand the diagnostic process that led to the decision making, to proceed with the surgery and the patient's concerns and fears. Surgical cases could be challenging. No two surgeries are alike. The technical aspect of the surgery was dependent upon the type of the disease, and the surgical findings. It was incredibly satisfying to see the patients doing well after successful surgical procedures. Most of the patients were cured entirely after removing the diseased organ. We had excellent surgeons, and each of their surgical techniques was subtly different. As residents, we picked up the best surgical techniques from each physician and made them our own.

OB-GYN physicians, as women's health specialists, we have the privilege of seeing women from the teenage years to the senior years, dealing with all the transformational phases of the women's lives. Obstetrics, gynecology surgery, and women's health was all part of our residency training.

Friends and Mentors

During my first year of residency, I was shy and talked very little. One person who got me out of my shell was my co-resident, Dr. Elmertha ("Mert") Burton. We were the only two female residents in the OB-GYN program that year. She was everything that I was not. She was an African-American woman, beautiful, confident, very sure of herself, and never hesitant to express her opinion or to disagree with the attending physicians, when appropriate. I was surprised to see that the attending physicians were flustered, but not angry when she spoke out or when she disagreed and expressed her own opinion.

In India, I could never ask or question my superiors. As a consequence, during the first year of residency, I was shy, expressed myself very rarely, followed all the rules, and performed every task I was supposed to do without asking any questions. Mert and I were different, she was outgoing, and I was shy, but somehow, we clicked. She took me shopping and introduced me to restaurants, margaritas, and disco. I was becoming a part of America and loved every bit of it. We became good friends and had so much fun together. We stayed as friends until the end of our residency. She moved to a different institution for her practice, and we slowly lost touch as both of us got very busy with our own lives. I later heard she had moved to Mississippi in the 1990's, her childhood home.

The second physician who helped me was my program director, Dr. Henry Maicki. He initially was critical of my shyness and would say he was not sure if I would be able to speak up with any patient care concerns to the physicians. He made me uncomfortable with his comments, and I felt they were condescending. I tried to avoid him as much as I could, which was difficult to manage, as he was my program director. However, I was getting out of my shell at the end of my first year, and I started more freely expressing my opinions and patient-care plans. In the middle of my residency, Dr. Maicki became my staunch supporter. I was doing well in my residency and was also in the top 96th percentile in the national exam. He challenged me to be even better and would make dinner bets with me when we disagreed. He kept his word and took me out for dinner if I won the bet. I think that this was his way of boosting my confidence.

During my senior year of residency, he invited Vinay and me to his home for Thanksgiving dinner. As we all know, it does take a village to bring up and nurture a child; as a young woman, who came to a new country and entered a new culture, I succeeded because I was supported and nurtured by a village of physicians. They helped me to be part of a community. How generous of Dr. Henry (Hank) Maicki and his wife, Marlen Maicki, to invite us into their home for a family holiday. The Maickis' invited all the residents for summer barbecues at their home. We became good friends. Hank and Marlen invited Vinay and me to their children's swim meets and holiday dinners. We got to know his children, Sandy, Rick, and Henry very well and I would go on bike rides with them. I had the privilege of delivering two of his grandchildren. Hank and Marlen were the ones who introduced us to the more elegant things of American life and culture, like country clubs and the opera. Hank was my mentor and my partner in practice for 20 years, and we consider Hank and Marlen as our dear friends.

Dr. Connie Tubbs was one of my attending physicians and was the only female attending physician in the OB-GYN Department at Providence when I was an intern. She was tough and had very definite opinions. I was terrified of her. I am sure she had to be tough to be in a specialty that was dominated mostly by men. She stood her ground, and it was good to see all the male attending physicians treating her as an equal and with respect. Dr.Tubbs did not say much to me, either positive or negative until I successfully managed a couple of her patients during emergencies. That was the beginning of our lifelong friendship.

Baptism by Fire

One night during the middle of my second-year residency, when I was on duty, a patient was admitted to the labor and delivery unit at 34-weeks' gestation (i.e., six weeks early) with cramping. The pregnancy was her fifth, with a history of four previous cesarean sections. The higher the number of cesarean sections in a woman's past, the higher the risk of uterine rupture and abnormal placental location leading to bleeding abnormalities that can be life-threatening for both the mother and the baby. At that time, we used to admit any pregnant patients who arrived at the hospital and kept them overnight, no matter what their symptoms were. After an appropriate evaluation and exam, I determined that this patient not to be in labor. Dr. Tubbs prescribed Seconal, a sleep medication, which was the accepted method of treatment in the '70s. It was an unusually slow night, and there were no attending physicians available in the labor and delivery unit.

After midnight, I was resting in the call room when one of the nurses, Sue Tozer, woke me up and informed me that she noticed a large blood spot on this specific patient's pad. That got my attention. I got up immediately, and we walked to the patient's room, which was just four rooms down from where I had been resting. It took me only a minute to get there and evaluate the patient.

I was shocked to see the blood pouring from her like a fully opened faucet. One nurse, Ellen, was already in the room, drew her blood for type and cross-match to prepare for a blood transfusion, and started intravenous fluids. It was like watching a symphony as the two nurses worked together as a team. Other nurses came in to help, but no one was speaking loudly or running around. Everybody knew what to do, and we knew we had to move her immediately for a cesarean section to save the lives of both the mother and the baby. However, there was no attending physician available. Today, it would be so different as there is always an attending physician—on call, in-house, 24/7—to cover emergencies. I got on the phone with Dr. Tubbs to inform her, her patient was hemorrhaging, and she needed to come to the hospital immediately. Nursing staff notified the anesthesia department. There was a 24-hour certified nurse anesthetist coverage, but no anesthesiologist was available. The nurse anesthetist could administer general anesthesia to the patient. The pediatric resident on-call was notified to come to attend the imminent delivery of this premature baby.

Nurses had already moved the patient to the cesarean section room by the time I was done talking to Dr. Tubbs. After Pesti (do not recall the last name), the nurse anesthetist, administered the general anesthesia, she started the blood transfusion with 0 negative blood (the universal donor blood). Due to this life-threatening emergency, I could not wait for a full blood cross-match before transfusing blood to the patient. A rotating, first-year family-medicine resident, who had no surgical experience was on a call with me. He was the best I could do regarding a surgical assistant. I did not have time to be nervous; everything was going so fast; it was a real life-or-death situation.

I started doing the C-section with the help of the first-year family medicine resident. After cutting through the layers of the patient's abdomen, it was difficult to ascertain the cause of the bleeding as the uterus was dark and blue. I thought maybe blood could be seeping into the muscle wall of the uterus because of a separation of the placenta from the uterus. I somehow cut the uterus and delivered the baby, who weighed approximately 4 pounds and whose arrival was six weeks early. When I handed the baby to the pediatric resident, I heard the baby taking its first breath with a weak cry. In 1976, premature babies who were born six weeks early had very high morbidity and mortality rates. I was comforted to know that this baby had a fighting chance.

However, I was not sure why the uterus was blue as there was no visible separation of the placenta as I initially had expected. I had never encountered anything like this during my two years of training. Dr. Tubbs, who lived very nearby, arrived and came to the C-section room just after I had delivered the baby. It was such a great relief to see Dr. Tubbs' face and know that I was no longer responsible for making life-or-death decisions for this particular mother. Dr. Tubbs was a very experienced and competent physician, clinician, and surgeon. We were unable to separate the placenta, and so, to save the mother's life, we had to perform a hysterectomy. We realized that the placenta had grown through the entire muscle wall of the uterus— through the weak scar from her previous C-sections—and into the bladder that lies in the front of the uterus. Once the cramping began, it caused the scar to rupture and the blood vessels of the placenta to tear, resulting in a major hemorrhage. (Placental hemorrhage can cause a blood loss of 500 cc/minute—that is, about one-eighth of the total blood volume of the patient.)

It is an extremely rare condition when the placenta goes through the entire uterine wall into the bladder. I have seen cases where placenta invaded part of the uterine wall, but never through the entire uterine wall into the bladder. When it does, the diagnosis is placenta percreta. It was the only case of placenta percreta I witnessed in my entire 42 years of clinical experience. After all was said and done, both the mother and the baby survived and did well. The nurses did a phenomenal job, a perfect example of teamwork. We did everything right that night. The nurses informed me, it took us a total of seven minutes from the time that I walked into the patient's room to the baby's delivery.

Once the crisis was over, most of the discussions were around how we saved the mother's and baby's lives. There was not much about what the mother must have been going through emotionally while she was hemorrhaging, lingering between the life and death. We did not even think to address her thoughts, fears, and concerns for herself, for her baby, and for the rest of her children. Yes, we succeeded in helping her survive, but we failed in addressing her needs as a person. One of the shortcomings of the medical profession, even today, is that physicians are not often aware of the thoughts and emotional needs of their patients.

After that case, Dr. Connie Tubbs took me under her wings, supporting me, guiding me, and teaching me. After that case, we became fast friends and regular visitors at each other's homes. Connie Tubbs had invited my husband and me to many Thanksgiving and other holiday dinners. Connie's sister Jane was an excellent cook. The Cornish hens Jane used to make for Thanksgiving dinner were out of this world. Jane's pineapple upside-down cake was my favorite. Connie used to love to make tacos, and she would invite all her friends in the summer for a taco party. Connie and Jane taught me how to play poker. Connie brought a few of our women friends together as a group to play poker every other month. I remember those times with great fondness.

Connie was a strong woman with absolute convictions. I do not think she could have survived as the only woman, in a specialty typically dominated by men for so many years, without having been a strong person. She always lived on her terms, and she died a few years ago after the retirement in Arizona.

Changing Trends in Childbirth

During our training, in that day and age, we mostly focused on learning the clinical issues, managing the conditions affecting the pregnancy, labor, and delivery. We did not focus on the nurturing aspects of childbirth. We did not give any time or thought, for example, to reassure the patient or address any concerns she might have had for her or her baby's life while she was hemorrhaging. In the U.S., we did engage patients by informing them of their clinical diagnosis, and their treatment plans more than the physicians in India. We tended to tell the patient what was wrong with her and what we were going to do about it, but we did so from a very patronizing perspective, assuring the patient "it will all be okay" without addressing her concerns, or even finding out if she had any concerns. It was around this time that patients began demanding different experiences and approaches to childbirth, and the medical profession, though resistant, was starting to take notice. The baby-boomer generation was and has always been the change-makers. They were not happy with the status quo. Some women were getting frustrated with the rules and policies of the hospitals.

The main concerns of the patients were routine spinal anesthesia, forceps deliveries, and the separation of the baby from the mother for 24 hours even if there was no real evidence of any problem. Patients wanted to go through the childbirth classes to learn how to cope with the labor pains without anesthesia. They demanded their husband or family member to be present during the labor and birth for support. They declined soapsuds enemas. In 1977, there was one physician who accepted such patients, and we considered them strange and weird. In 1977 and '78 these childbirth demands became a movement. Dr. Henry Maicki, my program director, and mentor started looking at the growing movement of home births performed by lay midwives and alternative birthing centers in the hospitals. The first alternative birth center was started in New York in 1975 as a project to develop the certificate of need for such a center, under a special contract with Blue Cross-Blue Shield. After visiting the alternative birth center, Dr. Maicki was convinced and understood the need to offer a safe alternative birth center in Michigan.

We are all well aware that the status of a mother and baby can change very quickly, endangering the life for both of them. He was looking for alternatives for the subset of patients who desired to have a home birth like experience and give them the advantages of a safe hospital delivery. I observed how his approach to the birthing process began to change. Dr. Maicki started supporting more natural childbirth, performing fewer episiotomies, and trying to change the hospital policies to allow mothers to hold their babies immediately after birth.

Natural childbirth and bonding with the baby shortly after the birth was revolutionary at that time, and many physicians were against it. Jan Barger, a nurse who worked in labor and delivery, was a believer in and an advocate for natural childbirth and pushed for the physical bonding of mother and baby immediately after the birth. She had a baby in mid-1978 and demanded to have delivery as *she* planned. Jan asked for an exemption from the routine hospital policies. She had natural childbirth and bonded with her baby immediately afterward. I observed the contrast in mother's experiences between natural birth, and the deliveries in labor and delivery where we sedated the mothers with Valium shortly after the baby was born, and the babies were taken away to the nursery before parents got to see the baby. I started thinking differently about childbirth and how we were robbing most of our patients, from this beautiful, emotional, loving, and bonding experience with their baby. I stopped thinking that these patients were strange and weird.

Under the leadership of Dr. Henry Maicki, and the support of Dr. Krohn, chairman of our department, with the approval from Sister. Xavier Ballance, the CEO of Providence Hospital, the decision was made to start the Family Birthing Center (FBC) at Providence which was due to open in January of 1979. The FBC would provide an alternative birthing experience with the comforts of a home-like environment and the safety of the hospital and was *one of the first of its kind in the entire state of Michigan* and one of the fourteen of such centers in the country at that time. In fact, we had to get approval with a certificate of need from the State of Michigan to start the center.

Much work went on behind the scenes to start the FBC. Dr. Maicki was primarily responsible for getting the approval. Dr. Maicki was hired as director and Jan as head nurse and were responsible for marketing the FBC, through multiple TV and radio interviews, promoting the center, including question-and-answer sessions with the audience. The FBC could not have happened without the support and encouragement of Sister Xavier Balance, the CEO of the hospital, and Dr. Donald Krohn, the OB-GYN department chair. Delivering in the FBC was a revolution in childbirth, and almost all physicians were against it. It represented too big of a change, and the change is always hard. Sister Xavier became a close friend of mine later in her life. A great visionary, she was ahead of her times, super-competitive and a staunch advocate of women's health and issues that affected women and children. I am not surprised that she supported the FBC.

I was due to graduate in June 1978. Vinay and I had to decide whether to stay in Detroit or move out-of-state to start a private practice. I loved Providence Hospital and wanted to stay. To remain at Providence Hospital, I had to get an offer from one of the attending physicians as an employee or start practice on my own. This second option was not practical because I had no understanding of the business side of private practice. Vinay had a great offer from one of the multi-specialty practices in the local area.

Meanwhile, I had an offer from Dr. Gene Otlewski, one of the pre-eminent physicians and teachers in our department, to join him. I liked him a lot. He was very kind to me from the beginning of my residency. He was one of the most respected physicians in the hospital. He was fun-loving, debonair, direct and honest. During our residency, if we made a mistake, he would find us, wherever we were, and take us to a private room to teach us the right way. He was a real gentleman in every sense of the word and a phenomenal physician. I felt honored by his offer and accepted immediately. Dr. Krohn, Dr. Maicki, and many of my other teachers expressed their happiness that I had decided to stay. I knew I belonged at Providence Hospital.

June 30, 1978, was the last day of my residency. During the graduation ceremony, a few weeks earlier, Dr. Donald Krohn, chairman of our department, spoke about my shaky start and him giving me a one-year-only offer. He continued by saying how happy he was about his decision to accept me into the residency and how much they would have missed out on one of the better residents in the department. I was not sure if he knew what an impact those words had on me. I was very thankful for his kind words. It is difficult to explain the feeling of acceptance from the teachers you have so much respect for, especially for a young woman who had traveled all the way from India. Providence Hospital became my first real home in the U.S.

Early Years of My Practice,1978 – 1985

If we don't change, we don't grow.
If we don't grow, we aren't really living.
--- *Gail Sheehy*

On July 1, 1978, I joined Dr. Gene Otlewski in private practice. However, the month before that, June of 1978, the last month of my residency had been hectic, preparing for board exams, attending graduation parties and buying our first home. My husband joined a multi-specialty group with the same start date of July 1, 1978. I had mixed emotions, which included both fear and excitement. There was the fear of the unknown in starting a practice and the responsibility that went with it, as well as the excitement of starting a new chapter in our lives. So, I did not have time to give much thought to starting in private practice. I had some understanding of how the clinical side of private practice operated. At the end of my residency, after I signed the contract, Dr. Otlewski advised me to come to see pregnant patients in his office during my free time.

I started going to the office one half-day a week, saw a few patients, and at the same time got to know the office staff. By July 1st, I already had a few patients whom I was following who were due to deliver by August. Nonetheless, the first year of practice involved a significant adjustment. As an attending physician, I was in charge of making all the clinical decisions and patients placed their trust in me to make all the appropriate treatment plans. I no longer had an attending physician to fall back on as I had had in my residency, someone who would help me to make the decisions. We had a great department, and Dr. Otlewski, Dr.Maicki, and other senior attending physicians were always willing to offer any help I needed. It dawned on me that at the end of the day, I was responsible for the care and the final decision would be mine.

It was a tremendous responsibility and could be scary, no matter how much training I had. Another challenge was, I had plenty of free time. Developing a new practice takes time. I would see a few patients a day. I did not know what to do with the rest of the time. I missed the hustle and bustle of labor and delivery. Every day after seeing patients, I would go to labor and delivery to offer my help. Every Monday, Dr. Connie Tubbs was on call in labor and delivery. While she was waiting for her patients to deliver, she taught me how to play backgammon. I enjoyed that time with her.

I learned very early on in my practice how little we understand the complexity of pregnancy. It is indeed a miracle when a baby is born perfectly formed, with a healthy cry and, thank God; most babies are born healthy. We assume all babies are going to be healthy until the unexpected happens. Sometimes we are surprised by unanticipated poor outcomes. In spite of all the tests performed during the pregnancy to assure the well-being of the mother and baby, many times we do not have any clues of what traumatic events the baby had been exposed to, such as subtle infections, exposure to environmental toxins, and unknown maternal genetic issues or vascular diseases. One of the perfect examples we can relate in more recent times is the Zika virus. By the time we figured out the Zika virus's impact on pregnancy, many babies had already been born with abnormalities.

Only obstetricians understand the awesome responsibility involved in giving care to the pregnant mothers, weighing the health of the mother *versus* the health of the baby. Occasionally, we struggle to determine the optimal time to intervene to save the life of the mother and the baby. We, obstetricians, tend to question ourselves wondering whether we are providing appropriate care to ensure the optimal outcomes in very complex high-risk situations. Sometimes it comes down to having to make a judgment call, hoping for the best results.

Over the years, the additional stress resulting from potential lawsuits has genuinely impacted physicians' psyches and led to the practice of "defensive medicine." As a result, we perform more tests than what may be necessary, which always leads to higher costs in health care. Soon, these practices become the standard of care in all cases, even when, in some cases, there is no support or evidence for better outcomes. We, the physicians, fall into the practice of doing more frequent tests, believing we are delivering better care, and are surprised when the results do not meet the expectations. Our patients, themselves, have come to think that the more tests we perform, the better the outcomes they can expect. Patients are then understandably overwhelmed by unexpected negative results and are usually grief-stricken and may, ultimately, become angry. It is hard for the physicians, to admit to patients that they do not have all the answers. This tendency is both a part of our medical training and our human DNA. The communication gap between the physician and the patient could lead to the frustration and the misunderstanding, and in some cases even ensued with legal action.

There is so much more we do not understand about the complexities of the human pathology, more than what we do understand. It is very stressful when the patients file lawsuits, especially, when their care meets the required standard of care. Every suit takes a significant toll on every physician, more so on obstetricians dealing with two lives, the mother's and the baby's, which involve multi-million-dollar awards.

In spite of all such challenges, I have not seen many obstetricians who did not love their job. The pleasure, the delight, the joy and the profound satisfaction we get from delivering a healthy baby is compensation for the challenges and stresses of this unique profession.

.

T.T's Story: A story of crisis and grace

I was in awe of the patients who chose not to take legal action in spite of less than optimal outcomes for them or a family member. One of those challenging cases happened to me in 1978, just a few months after I started my practice. T.T was one of the patients I had followed during my residency in Dr. Otlewski's office. She was a professional, and we bonded. One Friday afternoon, during her routine prenatal visit, she mentioned that for the past week she had been feeling decreased movements of the baby. She was 35 weeks pregnant. Fetal heart tones were normal. During my residency, if the mother felt decreased fetal movements, the routine practice was sent the patient home if heart tones were normal. Just around 1978, the research showed, one of the subtle signs of stress to the baby can be a decrease in the fetal movements. Research showed that a new non-interventional fetal monitoring test NST(non-stress test) might help to establish the fetal well being.

I accompanied T.T to Labor and Delivery. I wanted her to have the non-stress test, a test, which confirms the health of the baby. During the monitoring, the test result was equivocal. In 1978, additional non-invasive tests for further evaluation of the baby; like biophysical profile, and the doppler flow studies were not available. The only test available was the oxytocin challenge test (OCT), which requires the intravenous administration of the drug Pitocin to induce contractions. However, because NST was equivocal and she was still five weeks early, I did not want to induce contractions without an absolute indication to do so. I kept her in the hospital overnight to repeat the non-stress test. A repeat test did not show any improvement.

At that point, I decided to induce contractions by giving her an intravenous drip with Pitocin. As soon as she had experienced a few uterine contractions, the baby showed signs of fetal stress. I performed an emergency cesarean section. The baby girl, A.T was alive but had a very low Apgar score. This baby did survive but showed significant signs of compromised health and the potential for long-term developmental delays. I could not imagine what the parents must be going through, the confusion, the fear, and the sadness, not understanding what had happened and why their baby was not doing well when they believed the pregnancy was progressing normally. It was tough to describe my emotions at the time, which included the feeling of letting the parents down. I dwelled on it for a long time, considering how the parents' dreams of a healthy baby had been turned upside down in such a short time, and the significant challenges their baby would face with no chance of ordinary life. Moreover, it was difficult to fathom what parents would have to endure for the rest of their lives raising her. I felt responsible that I had failed this patient and spent many sleepless nights thinking about what I could have done differently.

I consulted with many of my senior physicians, after the fact, about how the events had transpired. They all agreed with my care, but that did not make me feel any better. I had no explanation to T.T and her husband why their baby was so compromised. T.T met all the criteria for a healthy pregnancy. T.T was a healthy woman with no medical illnesses, had never smoked or even had a drink during pregnancy, and the baby had been growing appropriately, which suggested a healthy placenta. So, what was the intrauterine event that caused such a significant impact on this baby? Was the baby, in utero, exposed to multiple chronic incidents over many months during the pregnancy, or was this outcome caused by an acute event within a short period, just the week before?

Why? Why? Why? I had no answers. The pregnancy that had started in such anticipation of joy and love had instead brought enormous challenges and sorrow. It is very common for parents to question the fairness of it all and express anger. Why did their baby have such problems when they did all the right things during the pregnancy, especially when others have healthy babies in spite of smoking, drinking or doing drugs? I did answer all the questions they had regarding the events that had transpired. I tried to give support to these parents the best I could under the most difficult of the circumstances. However, I was a young physician then, and I am not sure if I was able to give them all the emotional support that they needed.

In spite of all the studying and training, I have learned that there is so much we do not know. The worst part of it is, no matter what the reasons are for such an outcome, it is a lifelong heartache for parents to see their child growing up unable to perform the simplest chores that we all take for granted. The profound grief and anger that parents experience are very understandable.

I was surprised T.T came back to see me for her second pregnancy. It takes tremendous strength for parents to see the same physician when their previous experience was so painful. Many patients choose different physicians to have a fresh start and not to be reminded of their last experience every time they visit the physician. So, when T.T came back to see me, she showed great strength and character by placing her trust and confidence in me and allowing me to provide care for her second pregnancy. The second pregnancy went exceptionally well. I kept a close eye on the baby by monitoring the pregnancy with tests because of the complicated previous delivery. I performed an elective cesarean section at full term and delivered a healthy baby boy. I was grateful to T.T for giving both of us the closure that we so desperately needed. She needed to know that she was capable of having a healthy baby and I needed the trust she placed in me to care for her second pregnancy. I wondered, why the second pregnancy was perfect, without any problems, while the first pregnancy had significant difficulties? What had changed? Since it was entirely agonizing for me not to have the answer, I could not imagine what it must have been like for T.T and her husband not to have the answers.

These were extraordinary parents, and I was blessed to get to know them. They never took any legal action, despite T.T's husband being a lawyer. Even if I had done everything I possibly could have done, they could have still chosen the path of legal action against me. Their choice not to sue me says a lot about their core values, strength, and character. Above all, they taught me the gift of generosity in the face of adversity. No amount of medical education, studying, or training could have prepared me for what I learned from these parents.

A New Concept: The Family Birthing Center

During my early months of practice, Dr. Maicki became the director of FBC. Jan Barger was hired as a head nurse to the FBC. He had many conversations with me regarding the plans for the FBC, which was due to open in January of 1979. Providence Hospital decided the Birthing Center would be free-standing, located in a different building from the inpatient building of Providence Hospital in Southfield. This other building, the Fisher Center, had no connection to inpatient services or labor and delivery. We wanted to make sure we were offering a valid alternative to both hospital and home births. Dr. Maicki and Jan Barger hired the nursing staff. The staff took over the handling of the details of making the FBC a home away from home for the parents and bought furniture for two suites. Each suite had a living room complete with a sofa bed and a lounge chair as well as a bedroom with a queen-size bed to comfortably accommodate the father and the pregnant mother, a small crib for the baby, and a lounge chair. Each suite was complete with an ensuite bathroom with a bathtub.

Patients who desired to have a natural childbirth in a home-like setting started to switch to Dr. Maicki and sometimes to me with the plans of delivering their babies at the Birthing Center in January of '79. We had strict eligibility criteria to deliver in the Birthing Center. Pregnant women had to be low risk with no health issues for either the mother or the baby. To be considered for a birthing center delivery, the woman had to agree to be transferred to labor and delivery in the hospital if any concerns for the mother or baby arose during labor. The transfer time from the Fisher Center to the hospital's labor and delivery department was 3-5 minutes (there were many dry runs before opening the FBC).

This new concept of FBC represented a total revolution in childbirth. Our ideas and plans were the antitheses of all the procedures and processes typically engaged in labor and delivery. Our patients were free to walk during labor and did not want to have a routine episiotomy or forceps delivery. Most important, they desired to hold their babies immediately after the birth and experience no separation from their baby. Many physicians and nurses had difficulty in making the transition to these new expectations of patients. In general, human beings, tend to have trouble accepting any change and are most comfortable in their entrenched routines. The difficulty in accepting change is no different in the medical field. It is hard to embrace change, and any progress tends to be very slow, but we can not achieve the progress without the very changes that we are so resistant to adopting.

All the attending physicians were very upset with the concept of the FBC and truly believed that the deliveries we were offering at the FBC would endanger both the mothers and the babies. They were not considering our guidelines, which would enable safe deliveries for low-risk patients with closer monitoring of the mother and the baby. Our patients were monitored more frequently than patients in labor and delivery. It was and still is unheard of to have one nurse caring for just one patient in the hospital. Under our stringent guidelines, the nurse monitored the patient's heart rate every 15 minutes during the active stage of labor and after each contraction during the pushing stage of labor. In the hospital's labor and delivery department in 1979, the monitoring of low-risk patients was not as frequent. We tend to get into a "comfort zone" of following the procedures and the treatments from one generation to the next, without asking any questions. Some people accept changes faster than others. It takes much convincing to change many physicians' ideas, to leave their comfort zones. Physicians have developed a sense of safety and security, believing that following the same practices they learned does no harm.

We were challenging the whole obstetrical-care delivery system and the decades of entrenched standards of practice, which led to uncomfortable feelings on both sides. The more I learned about the practices in the other birthing centers in the U.S., the more I felt that the processes we had had in place during my residency may not have always been the safest. We knew having a pregnant woman lying on her back, reduced the blood and oxygen flow to the baby because of the weight of the uterus causing compression of the large blood vessels, yet we insisted that a patient should lie on her back during the labor. Most healthy babies tolerated it. However, some babies with subtle compromises did not tolerate a pregnant mother lying on her back. On the other hand, when a baby's heart rate showed any signs of stress, we made sure the mother was turned on her left side to enable the uterus to shift from compressing the major blood vessels to help the baby's circulation. We administered oxygen by mask to improve oxygen flow to the baby. We understood the steps needed to help the recovery of the abnormal fetal heart rate changes. Somehow, we did not connect the dots that it may not be the safest practice to have a pregnant mother lying on her back during the entire labor. Likewise, we did not think about the impact of separation of the mother and baby for twenty-four hours, without the mother even get to see—let alone hold—her baby.

V.W's Story: Her Perfect Birth

I wanted to participate in the FBC deliveries, and I do not think I had any idea how doing so would significantly change my entire professional career. V.W made an appointment to see me, wanting to deliver at the FBC that was due to open in the next few months. She called the FBC staff to get a recommendation for a physician who would be interested in delivering her baby at the FBC. The nurses recommended Dr. Maicki and me.

She decided to see me because I was willing to perform deliveries at the FBC and she preferred a female physician. It was amazing to see how far the society had come in four short years for a pregnant woman to prefer an obstetrician who was a woman in a field that was dominated by men. She transferred her care from another physician in the middle of her pregnancy. She had been disappointed in her two previous delivery experiences in traditional labor and delivery at the hospital. She was very calm and composed in her demeanor, but very determined and expressed her desire to experience the joyful and the intimate childbirth with her husband's support, by him being right next to her during the labor and birth.

Our conversations included how she did not want an enema, to have her pubic hair shaved, to be given intravenous fluids or to have an episiotomy. Her requests undoubtedly represented several significant deviations from how I had typically performed deliveries. V.W wanted an experience of natural childbirth with no medical interventions unless one was necessary. I was getting comfortable with the ideas of no enema, no shaving, or no forceps. However, no episiotomy or intravenous fluids? We routinely started intravenous fluids to be prepared for any emergency during labor and to administer Pitocin immediately after the delivery of the placenta to prevent uterine hemorrhage. Similarly, we had learned that a routine episiotomy reduced the risk of prolapse of the vagina supporting the bladder and the rectum because it shortened the pushing stage during labor.

I started feeling some trepidations and concerns when I thought about her requests. With them came some self-doubt. Topmost on my mind were the concerns for the safety of the mother and the baby. However, I was learning to listen and did not dismiss her requests. Do we need intravenous fluids for every laboring patient? Should we replace intravenous administration of Pitocin with medication that can be administered intramuscularly, after the delivery of the placenta to prevent hemorrhage? In India, we used to administer an intramuscular injection of the drug methergine just before the delivery of the placenta to avoid hemorrhage. So, V.W and I agreed not to start routine intravenous fluid unless it was necessary, and I would administer methergine to decrease complications from bleeding. I also addressed her concern regarding the episiotomy. I told her my fears that without an episiotomy, there could be tearing and possibly a prolapse, weakening the vagina. V.W was very well-informed and well-read about childbirth and indicated she was willing to take these risks. I wanted to honor V.W's wishes, when feasible, while at the same time, steering her away from any plans that I felt unsafe.

The FBC received much attention in the hospital, and the community, with all eyes focused on us, and many physicians in the OB-GYN department were watching our every step, expecting bad outcomes. They genuinely felt these practices would be harmful to the patients and their babies, and Dr. Maicki, as the director of FBC and a respected physician in the department, was getting most of the resistance from the other physicians. We were going against the wind, and it was not easy. The medical community always feels threatened by change and is afraid of losing control. This fear of losing control has always been difficult for physicians because we are in the business of saving lives and there is a certain amount of ego that goes with it. The philosophy of "we know better" trumped any reasonable patient's requests. Safety was always our top priority. Dr. Maicki and the FBC team developed strict policies to ensure the safe deliveries in the Birthing Center. The very last thing I wanted to do was to perform unsafe practices that would harm mothers and babies.

V.W understood and accepted the need to agree to be transferred to labor and delivery should any deviation from the usual labor pattern, or an emergency developed. I realized most patients were reasonable as long as the physicians were willing to listen and work with their requests when feasible. Safety involves teamwork. I cannot overstate the critical role that the nursing staff played. Every one of them was very passionate about keeping the focus on the pregnant woman's wishes for natural childbirth with no unnecessary interventions and no separation from her baby afterward. The nurses initially hired had to have work experience in the labor and delivery. Most of them were mothers themselves. They felt most of the traditional routines and interventions were unnecessary and that they robbed the joy of childbirth from the woman.

In January 1979, the FBC finally opened to the public. Dr. Maicki and I each had one patient due to deliver in January. We were all hoping Dr. Maicki would get to perform the first birth in the birthing center. V.W was my patient who was due in January, and she went into labor first. She called to let me know that she was in labor and was on her way to the birthing center. I was naturally nervous, wondering and worrying about performing childbirth that was so different than what I was trained to do. Dr. Maicki was there as the director of the birthing center and as a part of the team. All the nursing staff was there and was very excited to be part of this historic change in performing childbirth.

V.W walked in with her husband and family, totally calm and unfazed by all the commotion around her. She was ready to experience the birth of her dreams in the free-standing FBC, Southfield, MI. I examined V.W and determined her to be in labor. The nurse listened to the fetal heart tones, which were normal. She did not receive any intravenous fluids or get an enema or get her pubic hair shaved. I was nervous, feeling butterflies in my stomach, worried about what if the birth did not go well and in fear of letting V.W down, as well as everyone who was involved and who believed in this philosophy of birth. I was surprised by V.W's calm demeanor, her total confidence in herself and her body to experience the childbirth of her dreams. She was not at all frightened by the revolution on which she was embarking, that was entirely changing how we thought about the birth.

The presence of Dr. Maicki and all the nursing staff helped me to stay calm. The nurse continued to listen to her fetal heart tones at appropriate intervals per our FBC guidelines during her entire labor, while V.W was walking or lying down in a position that was comfortable. The baby's heart tones were good. Everything was going as planned. V.W was coping with the contractions by practicing Lamaze breathing with the help of her nearby husband, who was coaching her. She emitted no screams and asked for no drugs during her labor. I was anxiously waiting.

The time had come when V.W felt the urge to push the baby. She was lying in the queen-size bed with her husband next to her. Appropriate pads were placed under her bottom to decrease the possibility of contamination and to contain the fluid and blood. She was about to deliver the baby in bed with no intravenous fluids, no spinal anesthesia, no stirrups holding her legs up.

I was there only to support the mother and only act if and when my expertise was needed. As I watched V.W's-controlled pushing, I was thinking how much it must hurt as the baby's head stretched the vagina and the perineal skin. What a control she had! She appeared to be in "a zone." That was the first time I saw and understood the control of mind over body. That kind of power never ceased to amaze me, no matter how many times I witnessed it during all the years of my practice.

The nurse supported her bottom with warm compresses to avoid the tearing as the baby approached crowning. I did not perform a routine episiotomy, nor was there any reason to use forceps. I felt like I was standing naked, stripped of all my training. The mother was in control.

As V.W's baby crowned, I put my gloves on and gently delivered the baby's head with the help of V.W's slow, gentle pushes with her husband support, sitting right next to her. She had the full view of her baby's birth, watching it in a mirror. I suctioned the baby's mouth and delivered the baby's shoulders and the rest of the baby boy, placing him immediately on her abdomen as we heard his first cry. Even today, it is hard to describe the parents' emotion. Tears of joy were running down their faces while they gently rubbed the baby's back. Feeling the warmth of his mother's skin, the baby slowly opened his eyes. Bonding had begun the minute the baby was born. There was no whisking the baby away from the mother, and no drugs were used to sedate the mother. I clamped the baby's umbilical cord, and his father cuts it. It was a revolution in childbirth, first of its kind in Michigan.

This birth experience was a world apart from what I had experienced with the deliveries in the labor and delivery unit. The next step was to deliver the placenta. Immediately after delivering the baby, we used to routinely remove the placenta manually by inserting our hands into the uterus to separate the placenta from the uterine wall. In the FBC, we allowed time for the placenta to naturally separate, and when the patient felt mild cramping, she pushed the placenta out. I checked the placenta to make sure no remnants were missing. A methergine injection was given intramuscularly to prevent excessive bleeding from the delivery.

Everything had gone perfectly. There was much attention from the media. Robbie Timmons from Channel 7 interviewed V.W, Dr. Maicki, the nurse Jan Barger, Sister Xavier and me about the birth experience. V.W was a perfect person to be our first patient in the FBC. Given her non-assuming personality, her intent focus on having the natural childbirth, and her lack of interest in indulging in the celebrity nature of such an event made her the best person for this honor.

Now I had experienced, firsthand, the remarkable differences in the birthing process and its emotional impact on the parents between the standard labor and delivery and the FBC experiences. I began having more patients with a desire to deliver at the birthing center and the willingness to follow the stringent rules allowing only low-risk patients to ensure the safety of the mother and the baby. There were a few patients who wanted to deliver their babies at the birthing center, worried that the rules might "risk them out" of the experience that they so desired.

In the beginning, I was worried about some aspects of delivering the babies at the birthing center. I liked the natural childbirth experience we offered to the parents, but, at the same time, I had concerns and doubts if we could manage any necessary patient transfers to labor and delivery in case of emergency without any harm to the mother and baby. This concern weighed so heavily on me; once the patient called me to let me know that she was in labor, I would hurry and arrive at the hospital around the same time as the patient. While it might have been an overly cautious response, the practice of being with my patients for their entire labor experience helped me to bond with them. I was in awe of my patients' willingness to take responsibility for their childbirth choices and face criticism from their families and relatives, especially in cases of less-than-optimal outcomes.

What made a difference at the FBC was our exemplary teamwork. We had some of the best nursing staff led by the nurse manager Jan Barger and Mary Lou Longeway (Jan Barger moved to Chicago within a couple of years after FBC started), who were very passionate about their work and were the best patient advocates. As time went on, we had to transfer a few patients to labor and delivery for abnormal labors or abnormal changes in fetal heart tones. The transfers went well and resulted in good outcomes for the mother and the baby. Moreover, every time, we worked "against the tide" and succeeded, I felt a sigh of relief! As time went on, I became more comfortable and truly enjoyed delivering the babies at the birthing center. I remained with the family after the baby was born and witnessed the importance of the bonding between the mother and the baby and saw how the baby naturally latched onto the mother's breast. I held the baby and was often a part of the family pictures.

The bonding between the families, the nurses and the physicians at the FBC was so unique; we felt we belonged to one big family. Some of those relationships lasted a lifetime. All the mothers due to deliver in the birthing center attended natural childbirth classes, toured the FBC, and agreed to accept the strict birthing center policies. At that time the usual post-delivery stay in the hospital for a vaginal birth was five to seven days. Mothers at the FBC went home within six to twenty-four hours after childbirth. Follow-up protocol was for a nurse to call the family daily until the home visit on the third day to check both the mother and the baby. Nurses made more home visits if there was a medical concern or a need for emotional support. We provided the recommendations of a few pediatricians, who supported the idea of early discharge and were willing to see the baby within a couple of days after discharge to ensure they were doing well. Mothers were free to call the FBC nursing staff at any time of the day or night with any questions. The support families received from the nursing staff was phenomenal. Our patients felt we had their back. The success of the FBC involved true teamwork between the physicians, the nurses, and the patients. Our focus at the FBC was on the parents, aiming to make their experience both nurturing and safe.

From the beginning, there was mistrust between the FBC and the labor and delivery staff. L&D staff thought the birthing center patients were weird, that the care in the birthing center was suboptimal, and the nurses were not helping the patient understand the need for intervention when necessary. For their part, the birthing center staff believed the labor and delivery staff did not understand how to help this subset of patients achieve their need for a spiritual and emotionally satisfying birthing experience. I felt, we served the patients best, when the staff from both sides worked together and looked at the strengths of the other, with the focus on a safe *and* emotionally nurturing experience. Most of the physicians felt, and continue to feel, the same level of distrust in the care delivered in the FBC. Only a few of us loved delivering the babies at the birthing center.

The "V-BAC" Story: From Repeat Cesarean Section to a Vaginal Birth

During my residency, we learned that the uterine scar from a cesarean section would rupture during the labor of subsequent births, leading to morbidity or mortality of the mother and the baby. So, we all practiced by the dictum "once a cesarean section, always a cesarean section," meaning that once a woman had had a cesarean section, she would have another for each subsequent birth. Moreover, it is true if the uterine scar ruptures, it could result in significant compromise to the baby and the mother. Before performing an elective cesarean section, we made sure the baby's lungs were mature by aspirating and testing the amniotic fluid (i.e., amniocentesis), but amniocentesis, itself, has some risk of harming the baby.

Dr. Maicki had a patient who had had a previous cesarean section but who expressed her intense desire to have her husband present at the birth of their child. At the time, our hospital policy was not to allow a husband to be present at the cesarean section delivery. Dr. Maicki made a special request to the hospital administration and to the physicians in the department of anesthesia to allow the husband to be present at the birth, but they denied his request. Since the patient wanted her husband to be present at the birth, she insisted on trying a vaginal birth.

However, she was also scared of attempting a vaginal birth given the potential risk to the baby's life. It was hard for me to understand or explain to any physician, or to any person, why one wants to take the chance of risking her baby's life to have her husband present at the birth. Just around that time, in 1978, there was an article published in a reputable journal about the outcomes of accidental vaginal births after cesarean sections in Texas. Most of these births were members of the Latino population who were crossing the border to have the baby in the U.S. These mothers who had a previous cesarean section arrived at the hospital at the last minute, completely dilated and ready to give birth. The published paper reported many such deliveries with excellent outcomes.

Dr. Maicki read the article and decided to support his patient in trying a vaginal birth after her cesarean section, known then as a "VBAC" ("vaginal birth after cesarean"). Because the department of anesthesia declined to administer anesthesia if the husband were present at a cesarean birth, Dr. Maicki asked me if I was willing to provide spinal anesthesia to his patient, if she needed a cesarean section. I agreed to do it, so her husband could be present for the birth. We used to give spinal anesthesia to all our patients during vaginal births, so I had the privileges to administer spinal anesthesia. The administration and all the other physicians were all anxious and agitated by this decision.

Finally, the patient arrived in labor, with contractions, at the labor and delivery unit. I could not imagine the anxiety the patient felt after having made this monumental decision and taking on such a huge responsibility for her baby's life. Dr. Maicki stayed with her during her entire labor, all night, to ensure that both the mother and the baby were doing well. The patient, however, made no progress and had dilated to only two centimeters by the morning. Dr. Maicki called me to let me know the status of the patient and that he had decided to perform a cesarean section. He needed me to come in to administer the spinal anesthesia for her husband to be present at the birth. Both the mother and baby were stable.

It took me about 25 minutes to come to the hospital. After I arrived, nurses transferred the patient to the cesarean section room. As she was being helped to move on to the table, the patient stated she felt the urge to push. An examination revealed she was completely dilated and was ready to have the baby. She did have a vaginal birth with her husband present and with no anesthesia. My services were not needed, after all, but I was a witness to the first VBAC at Providence Hospital and one of the first few in Michigan.

There were very few physicians who performed VBACs. Dr. Maicki, another physician from Hutzel Hospital and I used to do most of the VBACs in the tri-county area. In the early years of doing VBACs, we noticed many patients would not progress for a long time; but would make progress and deliver vaginally, after we made the decision to do a cesarean section. During these years, I came to understand the burden on the mother after having made this most difficult decision against the recommendation of the medical community with very little support from the family members and the relatives. Going against the standard recommendations led to anxiety, which created negative feedback, inhibiting them from making progress in labor. Once the decision was made to perform a cesarean section, the mother felt the relief and no longer had to carry the burden of responsibility for her baby. The reduction in emotional stress eventually helped her labor to progress and allowed her to deliver the baby vaginally. I learned how negative biofeedback could influence our clinical outcomes. Within a decade, after a large body of evidence had accumulated, weighing the benefits and the risks of a VBAC versus a repeat cesarean section, VBAC became the standard of practice.

As my practice got busier in the second half of the first year, more and more of my patients were requesting natural childbirth. Even in the labor and delivery, Dr. Maicki and I allowed our patients to try ambulation, different positions during labor, and to birth in the labor room without moving the patient to the delivery room. No enemas! No episiotomy or forceps delivery unless indicated. The nursing staff, though uncomfortable at first, did begin to help the patients per our requests, albeit with reluctance. As nurses spent more time with the patients, they started noticing the advantages of ambulation and of being in different positions during labor. Nurses became the early converts to change. Of course, some nurses were not convinced and may never be.

Dr. Gene Otlewski had been very good to me. He visited the FBC for the very first time the day after the first birth, but only because of my participation. I appreciated his support for me, while at the same time, I understood his discomfort with the FBC practices, which were so different from the methods he believed. I respected him both professionally and personally as a physician and a person. His wife had paralysis from the complications during pregnancy. I admired how caring he was for his wife. He always brought her to all the department parties and made their situation look very ordinary. They adopted two children: a daughter and a son.

We were establishing a personal relationship at this time as well. Dr. Otlewski and his wife invited my husband and me for dinner and took us to the Fisher Theatre to see the musical "Show Boat." That was the first time we had ever gone to any live show. It was fascinating to see this story told through beautiful music. I have always been so glad that Dr. Otlewski introduced us to this art form and some of the subtler aspects of Western culture. Since that first show, I fell in love with the musicals so much that I do not think I have missed too many popular musicals since.

My Mentors' Generosity

As the first year of my practice was coming to an end, I had to make a decision. Dr. Otlewski was expecting me to continue for another year before I became a partner in his practice. My dilemma was how to tell this decent man, an excellent physician, and one of the leaders in the department and the hospital, that I was having second thoughts about continuing to practice with him. He was one of the very best traditional practitioners and believed in all the routine interventions from which I had moved away. In spite of my great respect for him, in the long run, I knew the differences in our beliefs and the processes related to the labor and delivery could create frustration and lead to my unhappiness. Of course, I also had to consider the challenges of starting a new solo practice. I had no clue how to go about it, and it would be a significant financial and administrative undertaking.

However, ultimately, I knew that going solo was the right thing to do. I talked to Vinay about it, and he supported me, wanting me to be happy. I did speak to Dr. Maicki about my fear of starting a solo practice. He, as always, reassured me that he would support me, and he asked his recently retired practice manager to help me until I got my new practice organized. Finally, I mustered the courage to talk to Dr. Otlewski and inform him of my decision not to continue with him in the same practice after the year ended. I explained to him the reasons why and that I had too much respect for him to stay under these circumstances.

I will never forget how gracious and kind he was in response. He asked me what my plans were, and I told him of my plans to start a solo practice. Not only did he extend his good wishes to me, he even asked me if I would be interested in covering his patients when he was on vacation. He indeed was a gentleman, and I believed he said all of that to make me feel better. He never once was critical of my decision or me, nor did he ever talk about me in a negative way to the members of the department.

Several years later, his wife passed away, and a few years after his wife's death, he married his second wife, Sharon. They were perfect for each other, and I could see how much they enjoyed each other's company. We became good friends. Later, they moved to a Victorian house on Harsens Island. My memories of him are still vivid to this day. I remember seeing the pictures of him fishing as a young man, on a horse at a ranch later in life. Sharon was an excellent cook, and I think of the joy he had on his face when having a good meal. He sent his daughter-in-law to me for maternity care, and I had the privilege of delivering his grandchildren.

In spite of all the challenges he had to face very early on in his life, he lived life with passion, and loved everything, whether it was playing golf, playing cards, or riding a horse in his '70s. He never hesitated to take on new challenges including learning modern computer systems. In his mid-seventies, he suffered a brain hemorrhage while playing cards and died from it. I was one of the few who spoke about him during his memorial service and expressed my appreciation of this man who was larger than life. How he was able to take the challenges of his life in stride without missing a moment of the joy life has to offer, and always with a little smile on his face and a twinkle in his eye. He was indeed a gift in my life for all that he had taught me about medicine, of course, but really, he showed me even more about life. Gene Otlewski is one of my heroes.

Solo Practice

On July 1st, 1979, I started my solo practice. A couple of months before that had been hectic. We sold our home and bought a condo. The profits from the sale were used to start my new practice. I leased office space in the Advance Building in Southfield. My husband helped me to buy second-hand office furniture and tables, and we hauled them in a U-Haul truck. Virginia, Dr. Maicki's ex-office manager, helped me hire my new staff. I recruited two women, a front-desk receptionist, and a registered nurse. I decided to hire a nurse rather than a medical assistant. Most physicians did not hire nurses because they were more expensive than a medical assistant. I felt having a nurse would provide an excellent benefit to my practice in the long run, because of the superior patient support they could offer, which would be of great help to both me as well as my patients

On the first day in my new office, I was able to see quite a few patients, and in the midst of it, I realized we had no trash cans. Oops! Starting practice was an exciting experience from which I learned a lot. Perhaps, most important, I learned not to back away from taking on new challenges and opportunities even when they made me uncomfortable. In time, I learned how to run a medical practice, and that served me well for the rest of my career.

My practice soon became very busy, and a lot of nurses and resident physicians came to me for their personal OB or GYN care. I was blown away by their support. I was very busy with the deliveries in both the FBC, as well as in the labor and delivery unit. I was on call day and night and delivered every one of my patients. I developed special bonds with my patients and them to me. There were nights, I am sure I was tired, but I cannot explain the joy I felt being part of the childbirth process, and I was very protective of each of my patients. I was enjoying my practice.

N.G's Story: A Story of Perseverance

One of the patients I bonded with, was N.G. I met N.G through her fiancé after I delivered his sister's baby. N.G was a violinist who played in Michigan Opera Theatre Orchestra, and her husband was a young engineer. She made an appointment to see me to discuss her unexpected pregnancy and how she and her husband had decided not to have children and wanted a termination of the pregnancy. I informed her that while I did not perform abortions, I would not judge anybody who chose that route. However, I went on to say the decision could be very emotional, regardless of whether one takes a "pro-life" or "pro-choice" stance and at the end, I hoped it was the right choice. I did say to N.G if she were to choose to terminate the pregnancy, she may feel the unexpected emotions of regret and she should not to be surprised if she experienced the afterthought of wanting to have children. I advised her that this could be a traumatic event and she needed to think through before she made the decision. I provided her with the recommendation of a physician if she chose to go through with it.

A few months later, she came to see me and said if I would be surprised, to know that if she had decided to get pregnant after all that transpired. I said, I was not surprised and was pleased to see her ability to change and listen to her heart. That is how we started our journey together.N.G is very intelligent, attractive, and pleasant to talk.

N.G did get pregnant. During one of her visits, around the middle of her pregnancy, she expressed her worries concerning how her mother had lost a baby at 32 weeks from pre-eclampsia. Pre-eclampsia happens to be one of the most common diseases that affect the pregnancy, with the signs of high blood pressure, protein in the urine, and edema. It is a vascular disease that can affect the circulation of all essential organs in the body as well as that of the placenta, which is vital to the baby's well-being.

Though most patients with pre-eclampsia have good outcomes, in rare situations, a severe form of pre-eclampsia can lead to seizures, sometimes even resulting in mortality of the mother and the baby. I found it not uncommon to hear patients express their fears during pregnancy, especially after listening to the others' experiences, most of them being negative. I understood her worry and concern, this being her mother's experience, and I reassured her that her pregnancy was going well. During her prenatal visit at 32 weeks of pregnancy, which happened to be a Wednesday, she had a mild elevation of blood pressure at 130/80 (normal for pregnancy being 120/80). However, she did not spill any protein in her urine, did not show any swelling of her feet, but her nose was slightly shiny suggesting a possible swelling of her face. I listened to the baby's heartbeat. Everything appeared to be well with the baby. N.G was thin and had a small build. I was always worried about even a mild elevation in blood pressure in lean women with a slight build, with no other signs and symptoms, as a possible sign of early pre-eclampsia.

I discussed with her that because of the mild change in her blood pressure, I wanted to monitor her closely and would like her to come to see me in two days, on Friday of the same week. The next morning, Thursday, I was at the hospital.N.G called me to see if she could see me that day. She was not feeling the baby move much, and her husband was leaving on a business trip Friday. I told her to come to the hospital so that I could evaluate her and the baby.

When she arrived, during the evaluation, we were not able to hear the heartbeat, confirming fetal demise. N.G's blood pressure was high, she was experiencing abdominal discomfort, and she felt that her abdomen was very tight. I realized that she had full-blown pre-eclampsia and most likely total placental abruption, which means there had been a complete separation of the placenta from the uterine wall, leading to fetal demise. Abruption is one of the conditions we cannot predict, no matter how carefully we monitor a pregnancy because of its sudden nature in onset.

As one could imagine, it was not an easy task for me, ---myself in disbelief of the findings, ---to muster the courage to explain to the parents — N.G, and her husband—that their baby was no longer alive. One of the worst moments in obstetrician's life is when the physician has to inform the parents that their baby is not alive. They had no time to absorb this shocking information or to grieve because N.G was very sick. She had minimal urine output suggestive of kidney involvement from the severe pre-eclampsia. I started her on the drug, magnesium sulfate, to prevent seizures, as well as Pitocin to induce the contractions, which would eventually enable N.G to deliver this baby.

During this period of waiting, I was in the head nurse's office crying, thinking about what had transpired, wondering how this could have happened. I was worried for N.G Her husband, who was walking by, saw me and gave me a big hug, comforting me by saying that it would be okay, and we would get through this together. How could he be so kind to me, the physician, while he was going through the grief from the sudden news of the loss of his baby and while being worried sick about his wife?

I have always wondered if I would be able to be as generous as he was if I were facing the same situation. I hope so. The kindness and courage of people are all around us when things get tough. It is up to us to open our hearts and learn to "pay it forward." On that day, that hug taught me more than anything we could have said to each other.

N.G's condition stabilized. I felt so unkind to put her through the labor or a cesarean section for a baby who was not alive. However, it was the right medical decision to induce labor and deliver the baby to cure the pre-eclampsia and save N.G's life. Her cervix was not responding to the Pitocin. Unlike today, we had no drugs to ripen the cervix. I decided to perform a cesarean section to deliver the baby. During the cesarean section, N.G's uterus looked blue, suggesting that the bleeding caused by the separation of the placenta had seeped into the muscle wall of the uterus. This condition is called couvelaire uterus.

Couvelaire uterus prevents the muscle wall of the uterus from contracting after the delivery of the placenta, which can lead to life-threatening hemorrhaging. After I delivered N.G's baby, I noticed her uterus was slow to contract, which would have led to significant bleeding, so I was very close to performing a procedure that ties off the blood vessels which supply the blood circulation to the uterus. If unsuccessful, my other option would be to do a hysterectomy to save her life. The thought went through my mind that she would never have children if I had to perform a hysterectomy, and this would be after all that she went through in changing her intention to have children. After giving additional drugs along with the Pitocin to contract the uterus, the uterus responded. My team completed the cesarean section with much relief that N.G was stable and that we had been successful in saving her uterus.

During the most devastating experiences, we tend to look for the things we have to be thankful for and find rays of hope for the future. Saving the uterus gave all of us that ray of hope for the future, that she would have the opportunity to be pregnant again and have children. N.G and her husband grieved appropriately, drawing the strength from each other and their families. I could never get over the fact that both N.G and her mother lost the babies to pre-eclampsia at exactly 32 weeks of pregnancy, which was another evidence of how much we do not understand. I learned not to explain what is beyond explanation, but to accept it. N.G was sad but not bitter throughout this devastating experience. Having a mother who went through a similar experience must have been a great help. Who else would understand her pain of losing the baby better than her mother who went through the same experience?

N.G, in general, is a very positive and forward-looking person. N.G got pregnant two more times, and I was delighted to be part of delivering two very healthy babies: a girl and a boy. Both have grown up to be responsible adults and are doing well. When I delivered her first healthy baby, her husband drove all the way to my home to bring a case of wine and sit with my husband, as I was not home. N.G's husband let my husband know how much they appreciated me. I only did what I was supposed to do, and, in my mind, that was my duty. I was not sure what I did to deserve their unconditional affection, but I was genuinely humbled by their generous hearts, their spirit of giving to the others, in both happy and sad times. N.G's husband's hug and his visit to my home were a clear reflection of this spirit. I hoped I would be like them if I faced such challenges in my life.

N.G had experienced many ups and downs in her life. She was diagnosed with early breast cancer when she was young, still in her 40s. She received appropriate treatment and survived the breast cancer, only to discover a few years later that she had non-Hodgkins lymphoma. She underwent chemotherapy with excellent results. Very early on in life,s he had gone through the loss of a baby and survived two cancers. She faced these challenges with tremendous grace under pressure and with a positive spirit, not giving up her zest for life.

However, she was at a crossroads in her marriage. Unfortunately, the husband she loved and the only man she had dated before her marriage became an alcoholic. She tried to cope with it to keep her marriage and family intact. We were close, and every time I saw her, we reminisced about our journey together. It was on one of those visits that, for the first time, she mentioned how sad she had been for many years and what she had been going through with her alcoholic husband. He was at the point where he was unable to care for his wife on an emotional level, but he was still able to hold on to his job in spite of his significant alcoholism. N.G told me he had refused to get help. I felt terrible for N.G, who was silently suffering while showing a smiling brave face to her family and friends. I was equally saddened to hear about her husband, the man who had, at one time, cared deeply about others. I remembered how he had consoled me with a hug, despite his deep sadness at the time of losing his first baby, and how he had visited my home to share the joy of the birth of his second baby.

Unfortunately, anyone who is genetically predisposed to the dependence on alcohol or drugs is vulnerable to these addictions. All these years, I had not known anything about what N.G was experiencing in her life. I thought she and her husband were one of the best married couples, a couple that would be able to overcome any obstacles in life together. No one knows what goes on behind closed doors, and I was stunned to hear of N.G's unexpected troubles in marriage. During our conversation about her situation, I encouraged her to consider divorce, which might be the only option that would allow her to avoid the emotional rollercoaster of sadness, anger, and helplessness in seeing her loved one going down the path of no return. She went home and told her husband of her decision to divorce him.

After the divorce, N.G, as usual, took her life in stride. This attractive, intelligent woman with such a zeal for life had no difficulty in finding dates. I occasionally assumed the protective role of a mother advising caution, though chronologically we are not that far apart. There were times she was frustrated with my recommendation of caution, but she was never in doubt about how much I cared for her. In the past few years, she has been in a relationship with a man she truly enjoys being with, and I have observed light and joy in her eyes every time she talked about him. I am truly happy for her.

During her last visit before my retirement, she was upset and was very emotional when she learned about my retirement. It was time to close a chapter of our lives and our long journey together. Through her tears, she thanked me for saving her uterus, which had helped her to have two children, and for being part of her life journey. I thanked her for being part of my life and the lessons she had taught me by the way she got up whenever she was knocked down with multiple challenges in life. Just in the span of 20 years, she had dealt with the loss of a baby, faced two cancers, and grieved the divorce from her first love, her husband. Few people I had ever seen could show such strength, courage, eternal optimism, hope, and faith when faced with so many obstacles in life. N.G is one special lady, and I will never forget her.

Over the years, I realized that the grieving processes are different for mothers who lose a baby before or at birth. In such cases, like in the case of N.G, there might be some closure, even though it might have left a scar for a lifetime. Whereas when a baby is born with a mental or physical handicap, parents, like in the case of T.T go through a long journey of hope and grief, hope the baby, in time, will be healthy and grief when there is no change. These parents experience additional pain when the baby is not improving as they had expected. It changes their lives forever. I have seen some amazing parents care for their mentally and physically challenged children with love and commitment, never complaining about the burden they bear. The wonder of it all was that the parents told me as many stories about their child with a handicap, as they did about their other children. I loved listening to those stories from the proud mothers and learned every child has a story.

Expanding Practice

My practice continued to flourish, and I was fortunate to have support from many young physicians and the nurses who would come to see me as patients and refer their friends to me. I was honestly honored and humbled by their support, but I was extremely busy working day and night without a break for a couple of years. One of the best resident physicians, Dr. Clarissa Cowles, three years my junior, expressed the desire to join me in my practice. We had bonded as residents, and I was her obstetrician during her second pregnancy and delivery. She was a mother of two boys. By the time she was ready to join me in January of 1982, I had a very thriving practice and was prepared to have an associate to share the medical practice and night call with me. Clarissa was one of the smartest resident physicians with an excellent bedside manner and great clinical and surgical skills to boot. She dove into my practice and was enthusiastic about delivering pregnant mothers at the FBC. Our style of practicing medicine was very similar, so patients were able to adapt well to her. In fact, patients loved her. Our practice expanded very rapidly and became one of the busiest OB-GYN practices at Providence Hospital.

Around 1983, Dr. Maicki decided to separate from his existing group and asked me if I would be interested in merging our practices. I felt honored that my mentor and my friend would invite me to join him in practice. Our practice philosophy was so similar that it made sense for us to merge our practices. Dr. Cowles, after an initial trepidation, agreed to move forward with a three-physician group practice.

In July of 1983, the three of us moved to a new office with high hopes for our future. Our merged practice flourished with the support of our office and nursing staff. In spite of our hectic schedule, our patients seemed to be satisfied with the support and care we delivered and appreciated the additional support provided by our dedicated nursing staff. One of the best decisions we made was to hire nursing staff instead of managing the practice with just one medical assistant. I believe one of the most important keys that led to our success was our nurse's availability to address all the concerns and questions of our patients. Our staff treated them with respect and kindness, forging trust and friendship, as well as long-term patient-practice relationships. Our patients believed we "had their back." However, life does not always proceed how we expect it.

In April of 1985, Dr. Clarissa Cowles, who had continued to develop as an outstanding physician, obstetrician, and gynecologist decided to stop practicing OB-GYN, due to personal reasons. We tried to encourage her to think thoroughly about her decision before she made it final. She chose not to postpone the decision, feeling it was best for her family. It was such a loss for her patients, for our staff, and for me. We were deeply saddened that she decided to leave. She had been so beloved by everyone who came in touch with her. Even many years later, her former patients would still inquire about her well-being. She practiced for only three and half years with us but significantly impacted her patients with her superior clinical care, as well as her genuine and down-to-earth bedside manner. After we said our good-byes to Clarissa, Dr. Maicki and I continued our joint practice. Clarissa was sorely missed.

Early-Pregnancy Loss

She wasn't just expecting a baby;
she was expecting the rest of their lives.
-- *Unknown*

In my experience, most couples spend a lot of time thinking and planning before they decide to become parents and start a family. The woman plays a more significant role in pushing to start a family. Sometimes the man wants to wait for an optimal time until they are financially secure, but the woman often worries about her biological clock ticking away with an increasing concern that her window of opportunity to get pregnant is getting smaller.

When a woman decides that she is ready to start a family, the excitement she feels in anticipation of getting pregnant and having children is very visual and palpable. Some women come for pre-pregnancy counseling, and others do not. Pre-pregnancy counseling is always advisable to learn about the genetic diseases that may require prenatal testing, routines of do's and don'ts, and best methods to reduce the risk to the fetus. Most women change their lifestyle to ensure their baby's well-being by avoiding alcohol and specific medications and by quitting smoking while they are trying to get pregnant and during pregnancy.

While she is trying to conceive, a woman goes through a monthly cycle of the anticipatory excitement of being pregnant, followed by a significant disappointment when she does not become pregnant. About 90% of the women get pregnant within the first year of trying. No matter how much a woman receives the counsel that it might take a few months to a year to get pregnant, most women expect to get pregnant the very first month that they try. The woman feels that if she and her partner are "normal," she should be able to conceive the very month she starts trying. It makes no sense to her why she does not get pregnant immediately. So, the anticipation soon becomes a concern tinged with the anxiety, thinking that something could be wrong with one or both of them.

We are now a society of planners, so it is not unusual for a woman to plan the month she wants to get pregnant and the month she expects the baby to be born to fit into the couple's schedule. Unfortunately, conception does not have any regard for one's agenda. Women have difficulty understanding that there is more to get pregnant than the presence of a sperm and an egg, and the fertilization does not occur according to the couple's timeline, or in a slot on their calendar. Women are postponing pregnancy because of their career choices. Once they decide to become pregnant, the emotional stress can be very intense until they conceived, constantly reminding themselves that the window of the biological clock was ticking away.

The minute the woman becomes pregnant, often the parents' dreams for their baby are unleashed, beginning with the birth of the baby to marriage and everything in between: birthdays, graduation, college, and so on. Against this emotional backdrop, when a couple goes through a miscarriage, the emotional impact and their grief may be more significant than their physician's perceived understanding of the couple's grieving process.

After a miscarriage, the first question a woman asks is if the outcome would have been different if she had done better with the diet or activity. She starts questioning everything she did or did not do regarding the food she ate, activities she was involved in or any medications she might have taken. The next question is will she be able to get pregnant again and what will be the risk of miscarriage in the future. As physicians, we tend to give a scientific explanation to the couple that the miscarriage is usually the result of an unhealthy fetus, so the miscarriage was unavoidable, no matter what she ate or what the activities were. However, for the parents, no matter what the reason for their loss, the miscarriage remains to be the death of their baby, and the lost dreams of their child. The intensity and the duration of the grief response to an early miscarriage vary from one woman to the next, and we are not always in tune with the patient's grieving process and its long-term emotional impact. Even though the physicians reassure the patient her risk of miscarriage for the next pregnancy would be the same as the first pregnancy; the patients continue to have the lingering doubts and feel stressed until they had a successful pregnancy and the birth.

F.F's Story: A Teaching Moment

Personally, I thought I understood how a miscarriage impacts a mother's emotions, who had already visually imagined her child's life the minute she realized she was pregnant. I responded to each loss by talking about the different stages of grief and by supporting the parents' grieving process. Subsequently, I saw that many of my patients did move on emotionally and had successful pregnancies. In spite of my understanding of the women's emotions tied up in the early pregnancy loss, I was surprised to hear how one of my patients, F.F, had felt about her miscarriage from more than twenty years ago. The week before I retired from my practice, I had a conversation with F.F We talked and reminisced about the past and her painful experiences with several miscarriages before she successfully had a full term pregnancy and delivered a healthy baby. I was taken aback when she said that every year on Mother's Day she feels sad and very emotional thinking about her lost pregnancies, wondering what each unborn child would have been if they had been born. I realized that it is not just the *immediate* emotional impact, but for some mothers, it is a lifetime of mourning, quietly carrying a hole in their hearts as they move on with their lives.

I do have to say, I never thought about what mothers could have been feeling many years after an early-pregnancy loss. Early miscarriages are not often a part of a regular conversation later on in a woman's life in the same way that the subject of a baby's death often is, maybe because of the high frequency of miscarriage. F.F 's conversation gave me the insight that no matter how early the loss is, for some mothers, it leaves an underlying layer of sadness for the rest of their lives, often wondering what might have been. Another teaching moment, at the very end of my professional career!

Having one miscarriage is extremely hard on any woman. When a woman has to go through multiple miscarriages, it is hard to imagine the level of grief fear and anxiety a woman feels with each subsequent pregnancy. Statistically, having one incidence of miscarriage does not increase the risk of miscarriage in subsequent pregnancies. Women who have had three consecutive miscarriages receive a diagnostic workup to determine if there is an underlying condition contributing to the persistent early-pregnancy losses. The most common cause of miscarriages is the presence of a random chromosomal abnormality. Other less frequent problems include inherited chromosomal abnormalities, hormonal imbalances, endometriosis, uterine abnormalities, inherited clotting diseases, advanced maternal age and lifestyle issues like drugs, alcohol, and smoking and other genetic conditions. We treated some of these underlying conditions, and in many cases, the treatment results in healthy pregnancies and healthy babies. Chromosomal abnormalities in either of the parents though rare present the highest risk for future miscarriages, and such a situation, understandably, leads to an emotional rollercoaster ride of decision-making.

W.D's Story: A Lesson of Hope, Strength, and Resilience

Many of us have different spiritual beliefs at our inner core, and often we do not know our strengths or how we would react when faced with a challenge. One of my patients showed me a spiritual strength beyond what I could imagine was humanly possible. W.D had come to see me for obstetrical care during her first pregnancy in the early-1980s. During those days, we did not perform a routine ultrasound in the first trimester of pregnancy, which, now, often used to determine the viability of the fetus. Once the pregnancy test was positive, we considered the pregnancy to be healthy unless the patient showed signs of miscarriage.

In the first trimester of pregnancy, W.D started having episodes of bleeding and ultimately had a miscarriage. As expected, W.D and her husband were very disappointed. The grief from the loss of a pregnancy is not any less, even if one understands that the most common cause of miscarriage is a random chromosomal abnormality and that the baby may not have been healthy if the pregnancy had continued.

After an appropriate grieving process, she and her husband decided to try again. Her two subsequent pregnancies also led to an early miscarriage. With three consecutive miscarriage, the toll on parents who desperately want a family significantly increases. Such parents eventually may be overwhelmed and fall into a depression for the loss of the pregnancies, and the uncertainty of their future to be able to have children. W.D was in her thirties and anxious to know if there was an underlying cause that had contributed to her three consecutive miscarriages. They felt relieved when I suggested testing them for chromosomal abnormalities first before I started more extensive testing. I expected the results to come back normal because in most cases they are normal.

So, I was somewhat surprised to receive the result of W.D's husband's test suggesting an abnormal chromosomal pattern with what we call a "balanced translocation." The outcome of a balanced chromosomal translocation is that the person's genotype is abnormal, but his/her phenotype--physical appearance and function--is normal. There are no other means we can recognize a person with an unusual chromosomal pattern unless we perform the blood test for karyotyping (chromosomal analysis). I asked W.D and her husband to make an appointment to discuss the results of their karyotypes. W.D's husband's test showed the type of translocation which carried a very high risk of miscarriage. Giving painful news is one of the situations that physicians agonize over. How does one reveal such information that could affect the parents' plans of having a baby forever?

When they were in my office, I informed them that I had received the test results. Then I told them that W.D's karyotyping was normal. Next, I communicated to them that W.D's husband's results appeared not to be normal. Finally, I informed them that this type of abnormal chromosomal pattern most likely was the cause of the miscarriages. On the top of that unexpected news, I also had to tell them that his kind of abnormality had a 75% chance of having an unbalanced translocation with each pregnancy, in which 100% of cases resulted in a miscarriage. Finally, I gave them some hope. With this abnormality, there was a 25% chance of having a baby with a balanced translocation, which would have a normal phenotype (normal function and physical appearance), but an abnormal genotype, like W.D's husband.

I went on to discuss their options, given the situation. Their first option was to continue to try to get pregnant with the hope that the next pregnancy would be a baby with a balanced translocation. The second option was for W.D to be artificially inseminated by a donor, so the baby would have shared genes from W.D The third option was to consider adoption. Of course, a fourth option was to remain childless. At the end of this discussion, I talked at length about the difficulty of the decision-making process that lay ahead, the stages of grief that one might experience with the new information they received. I answered all their questions, and offered my support to them, regardless of what option they chose. They were stoic and never broke down after learning this life-altering news as I had expected they would. I was not sure what their decision would be, but one thing I knew was that no matter what option they did choose, they are burdened with making a decision which has no easy choice.

I suggested they take the time needed to process through all the options and be clear-minded about their decision. W.D and her husband appeared to be a stable couple. W.D understood the situation and knew they would have to come to a shared conclusion about their plans for a family. On the one hand, W.D would have to physically endure the high risk of miscarriage and put her body, mind, and soul through this brutal experience of pregnancy and possibly miscarriage. Her husband, on the other hand, was the one carrying the abnormal chromosome. Any person who bears the burden of an inherited abnormal gene tends to be overwhelmed with the guilt and feel responsible for all the difficulties that they or their loved ones have to experience. While W.D's husband was not accountable for this abnormal chromosome, he could not, but feel responsible for what they both had endured in the past and possibly would have to face in the future.

W.D and her husband decided to continue to try to get pregnant with the hope that one day they would have a phenotypically normal baby. Fortunately, she never had difficulty in getting pregnant. She had three more miscarriages, for a total of six. With every one of these pregnancies, she would walk into my office with a quiet confidence that this one would be the one. I used to get very anxious and pray every time she came in for a pregnancy visit. I could not imagine how devastating it had to be to go through the pregnancy losses wondering if she would ever have a baby and what each baby would have looked like if the pregnancies were normal. I did not want to sway her decision or negate her need to have a baby, but I could not help and continued to give the gentle reminders of her other options. She was steadfast in her determination to keep trying, and I did not try to stop her. I am not saying she was not emotional about her miscarriages, but I never once heard W.D complain about her situation or despair about the future. At this point, I had seen thousands of women facing different challenges during my thirty-eight years of practice, but W.Dwas one of the few patients who never wavered or lost hope, not even once. Her hope, faith, and self-determination prevailed, and W.D and her husband eventually were blessed with three children. They are a unique couple, and W.D is a phenomenal woman.

S.E's Story: Understanding Loss and Grief

Women who are unable to have more children after the birth of their first child can feel more frustrated, not knowing the reason for secondary infertility, and consequently become more challenging for the physician to help adequately. S.E was one of my patients who had an uncomplicated pregnancy that resulted in the birth of a healthy child. Subsequently, S.E went through a series of pregnancies ending in miscarriages. After each miscarriage, she became more despondent. I performed all the recommended tests to find the underlying cause and was unable to find the etiology of her miscarriages. She was not only depressed but started showing the signs of being physically sick. I strongly advised S.E to see a counselor and a psychiatrist. She loved her only child very much, but she could not provide the best support to her child under these circumstances. She was a nurse by profession and had access to narcotics. To alleviate her emotional pain, she became addicted to drugs. S.E had been one of my favorite nurses, fun to be with, always brandishing a beautiful smile before all this happened. Seeing her go through such intense grief, suffering, pain, and addiction, which even affected her relationship with the only child she had, whom she loved very much, was one of the painful experiences I had to witness helplessly.

We, in our rational thinking, question how she could not see what was important, that is the child she already had in her life. Could she not overcome her grief with her unconditional love for her child? How could she go down the spiral of addiction? That is how we think when we are on the outside looking in, but we are not on the inside of her experience. In the end, it might have come down to the shock and inability to cope with the unrealized dreams of what S.E felt would have made her family complete. Not being able to have more children was out of her control and this led to intense grief and despair. Her emotions took over, she was suffering, and narcotics eased her pain, no matter how temporary the relief was. Everyone responds differently to pregnancy losses. Most go through the grief of a loss but can move forward, whereas, for the others like S.E, it is a life-long struggle for recovery and healing.

U.U's Story: A Contradictory Response to the Desired Pregnancy

Medicine turns out to be more art than science on more than one occasion, and sometimes outcomes defy the logic of science.

Many times, patients were unable to get pregnant for years, even after the infertility treatments. Then, I noticed, after all the infertility workup and treatments were exhausted and the parents finally decide to move forward, the woman would get pregnant, sometimes right after they adopted a baby. That defies science, and it is difficult to understand why they could not get pregnant for years when they had been trying all along. I used to jokingly say to my patients that God keeps more secrets than he lets me in on as a physician, to understand why things happen beyond the realm of explanation.

U.U was one of my patients who was trying to start a family. She got married in her late-'30s and wanted to get pregnant and have a baby immediately after getting married. She did get pregnant but had two consecutive miscarriages. Considering her age, I referred her to an infertility specialist. There is an increase in the risk of genetic abnormalities and miscarriage when women get older. After the two miscarriages and years of fertility workup, U.U was unable to get pregnant. When she was in her early '40s, her fertility specialist told her that she might never be able to get pregnant. She and her husband accepted the outcome and decided to move on with their lives and were content with the decision.

A few years later, at age 45, when she was least expecting, she became pregnant. Getting pregnant spontaneously at the age 45 was not a common occurrence, especially when one knows her chances of getting pregnant were bleak. When U.U came to see me, I expected her to be excited about the pregnancy and, understandably worried about being pregnant at the age 45. She was resentful that she had become pregnant after she had moved on in her life, accepting a life without children. U.U contemplated terminating the pregnancy. I was taken aback by her response, remembering how much she had wanted to have children, the miscarriages she had endured, and the infertility workup she had undergone just a few years ago. I realized, part of the reason for her unexpected response could be, she was worried about her ability to carry a healthy pregnancy and the risks for her and the baby.

I discussed with U.U the increased risks of diabetes and hypertension, due to her age, but she had been a very healthy woman, and pre-pregnancy health makes a positive difference in outcomes. Her baby had a higher risk for chromosomal abnormalities, and a test could be performed to determine the baby's status. I told her that it is okay to take a couple of weeks before making any decisions, so she would not have any regrets later. I informed her that if she chose to continue her pregnancy, I would be monitoring her pregnancy under very close surveillance. I was happy for her when she told me that she decided to have the baby. The baby's chromosomes were normal, and the pregnancy went well with no complications. She delivered a healthy baby girl. It was a heartwarming experience to see the beaming smile on U.U's face, her response to the relief that she was able to have a healthy baby.

During my career, I came to understand that a woman's dreams of a family are not confined to just having a child but include how many children would make them whole as a family. I have seen the disagreements between a wife and her husband about how many children will make them complete as a family. Most couples agree to have two children. Some together decide to have more children. However, sometimes the husband feels two children made his family complete. Fathers think more about what it takes to raise a child and the financial responsibilities that come with it. Right or not, men think and worry more about financial obligations. Whereas a woman feels her family is incomplete when she planned on having more children.

Disagreements between the couple about the size of the family is not a trivial issue. I felt the physician should not convince such a woman that she should be happy with the two children that she already has and should feel blessed for having two healthy children. If a woman plans on having more children, her family remains incomplete. Realizing that she will not have the number of children she planned involves a grieving process, too. Such women may experience the same stages of grief as women who miscarry. To experience the grief, one does not have to go through a physical loss; the grieving is equally intense with emotional loss. For some women, it is harder to recover and may require counseling to heal.

These were the teaching moments provided by my patients. Whether it was W.D's strength, resilience, hope, and faith in achieving her goal, or S.E's struggle with insurmountable grief, which led to her drug addiction, or

U.U's initial response to pregnancy with resentment, which she had so wanted just a few years earlier. These responses are not written about or learned from any medical textbooks. Just like our body's response is an enigma in some instances, our mind, the temple of our thought and emotions, became more mysterious to me.

I had to learn to readjust my thinking to understand some of my patients' responses. Loss, in whatever form it comes, has an impact on those who are experiencing it, well beyond our understanding. Such is life, with all its colors displayed differently at different times.

Middle years of My Practice 1985-1991

She was brave and strong and broken all at once.

--- Anna Funder

Our practice during the years of 1985-1991 was the most rewarding, and, at the same time, the most exhausting. After Dr. Cowles' departure, Dr. Maicki and I were very busy. Our practice was unlike any others. We preferred to attend all the births of our patients during the daytime but covered for each other during the night. Sometimes patients would end up waiting two to three hours for a ten-minute visit with a physician. The only reason I think the patients were willing to see us was for the personal experience we offered them during the pregnancy and the childbirth. We, along with the assistance of our nursing staff, provided our patients the support they needed and made them feel like they were part of the team.

The new generation of mothers decided to take control of their labor and childbirth from the traditionalists. Even many years later, many of my patients would emotionally mention, over and over, how wonderful their experience was when I helped them to participate in the final phase of delivering their baby, holding and guiding the baby out, while experiencing the emptiness of the uterus. At the time of birth, I thought it was a unique experience when parents participated in their baby's birth. However, I did not realize the lifetime impact of this singular event, and how it was one of the shining moments in the joyful memories of their baby's birth. I learned what is ordinary in a physician's practice may not be so routine to the patient and could have a lasting impact on her/his life, as either a positive or a negative experience.

For centuries, childbirth always was a life-or-death situation for both the mother and the baby, and many women and babies did not survive delivery. Medical interventions helped to increase the survival rates of the mother and the baby. Even now, in the majority of third world countries, mothers and babies lose their lives during childbirth for the lack of seeking health care or for the lack of access to health care. FBC created a unique hybrid model, combining the medical supervision in a home birth like setting, which helped my patients to have a safe, holistic nurturing birth experience. It was my patients who taught me about the holistic approach to birth—mind, body, and spirit.

Tests and technology help us to more successfully make the diagnosis and advance the treatment of many conditions that we could not have otherwise treated successfully. The availability of ultrasound during the early and mid-trimester pregnancy, blood tests to determine the pregnancy, and blood tests to screen for genetic diseases are just a few other examples of such helpful technology that have evolved beginning in the 1980s. These diagnostic tools help us diagnose life-threatening tubal pregnancies before they rupture, early pregnancy loss, fetal malformations (or the well-being of the baby) and pelvic pathology. In spite of such advanced medical technology in prenatal and newborn care, the U.S. still ranks 34th in the world in infant mortality.

Learning the appropriate time to manage the intervention and the non-intervention during the pregnancy and the birth is very challenging for the physicians. Like most physicians, I have always been for the advancement of medicine to help improve the human condition. However, not all interventions are safe, although their existence tends to give physicians a false sense of security. Evidence in medicine is a fluid condition and is continually changing. I have read, it takes an average of seventeen years for most clinicians to adapt and change to evidence-based methods from their original time of recommendation. As physicians, we tend to forget the importance of *learning* and *unlearning* as part of our collective conscience in advancing the human condition.

In 1987, eight years after the FBC came into being, a new labor and delivery unit was constructed to facilitate labor and delivery in the same room. The labor and delivery guidelines slowly evolved to include no routine enema, pubic shaving, spinal anesthesia or forceps delivery. Patients were able to ambulate while in labor. What was perceived as such a radical practice in the late 1970s would become more accepted by the late 1980s? Even if a patient experienced more interventions in labor and delivery, this still was a giant leap from where we had been ten years earlier.

Thirty years later the discussion about changing the practices in childbirth is still controversial. In the last few years, guidelines for childbirth practices are similar to what was advocated by the FBC, thirty years earlier. ACOG

(American College of OB-GYN) guidelines suggested that it is more beneficial for the mother and the baby; if the mother; does not have a routine episiotomy, does not push until she feels the urge even after full cervical dilation, and does not hold her breath during the pushing process. I heard some physicians, some of whom I respect, grumbling about these recommendations.

Of late, there has been research-based evidence that showed the significant health benefits of breastfeeding the babies, which had led to creating more baby-friendly hospitals. Physicians felt uncomfortable with the absoluteness of the recommendations, and some patients felt challenged by the stringent rules and the inadequate support system.

During my OB practice, most of our patients used to breastfeed their babies for six months to a year. Even these mothers, who were wholly committed to breastfeeding and made all the necessary preparations to do so during their pregnancy, still needed a lot of handholding and support during the first few weeks after the birth from the hospital nursing staff and my office staff. In the first few weeks, a new mother is challenged by the insecurities of being a mother, intensified by the added sleep deprivation, both of which may be exaggerated by postpartum hormonal changes. The uncertainty gives rise to many anxieties as a new mother wonders if the baby is okay and getting enough to eat, why the baby is crying, and why the baby is not awake enough or awake too much. During this intense period, often within the first month, mothers are more vulnerable to giving up breastfeeding.

First-time mothers who did not have the support found it challenging to breastfeed as they were adjusting to a new balance between the work and their new maternal responsibilities. Not all the mothers adjust the same way after the childbirth. Factors like a woman's personality, family background, and the level of family support play a role in how a woman responds to being a mother. Immediately after birth, it is more important than ever to have a woman giving support, encouragement and positive reinforcement, assuring new mothers that they are doing well.

In the early years of my practice, what we accomplished at the FBC still is a model for teamwork and patient-centered care, resulting in a nurturing environment created by the support of the family, staff, and physicians that go beyond the new mother's discharge. Women who chose the FBC were well-prepared and took responsibility gracefully, not just for the process of labor and birth, but to some extent, for the successful outcomes of that process.

G.G's Story: Grace Under Pressure

As an obstetrician who performed births both in the FBC and in the labor and delivery, I learned about the differences in patients who desired to have a birthing experience at the FBC. FBC patients were willing to take responsibility for their decisions and had a set of expectations before the birth.

G.G was a very healthy young woman who came to see me for care during her first pregnancy. Her pregnancy progressed well and met the low-risk pregnancy criteria to be allowed to birth in the FBC. When she went into labor, she progressed slowly but continued to make progress. It is not uncommon to have some labors that are longer than others, and it is normal to continue to monitor if the mother and baby are doing well. G.G delivered a large baby girl, who weighed 9 pounds. When the baby, E.G was born, she cried, but we noticed she had faster than normal respirations. I consulted a newborn specialist, a neonatologist, who decided to transfer the baby to the Neonatal Intensive Care Unit. Within 24 hours, the staff in the Neonatal ICU noticed the baby having seizure activity. The baby experiencing seizures raised an extreme concern, as it was possible that the baby had suffered from decreased oxygen during the birth process. However, the baby's heartbeat had been good during the labor and birth. I questioned myself and struggled to find the answers.

G.G came to see me for her six weeks' postpartum checkup. We talked about the birth, the status of the baby, the roller coaster of emotions she had been experiencing, and the uncertainty of the long-term prognosis for the baby. She said some of her family members were encouraging her to sue me for this less-than-optimal outcome, but she said she decided against it. Though it was difficult for me to hear her family's advise to sue me, I was not surprised by it. However, I was amazed by her strength and determination not to go through the legal route and to resist the pressure from her family members, despite her worry for her baby's future. She did not talk about her faith, but it appeared her decision not to pursue a legal option was mostly a reflection of her values and her commitment to being true to herself while trusting in God and hoping that everything would be okay.

Our relationship lasted for more than 30 years until I retired. I had the privilege of delivering four more children for her. I was fortunate enough to watch, E.G grew up with no residual effects from the seizure activity, she had experienced as a newborn. E.G earned two master's degrees and became a productive citizen in the community, was married and became a mother herself. E. G's healthy outcome is a perfect example of how much we do not understand about the cause and effect of trauma in pregnancy, labor, and birth, and how difficult it is to predict long-term outcomes. I have seen some babies with perfect Apgar scores who have developed learning disabilities. There is so much more to learn about the intrauterine environment and the role it plays in achieving the optimal outcomes.

G.G continued to be my patient until I retired. She is one of the most unassuming people I have ever encountered, who lives life from within a moral and spiritual center. I learned more about her when she and her husband decided to adopt a child with the emotional issues who was in a foster care. It was challenging to care for this emotionally-challenged child. The child is a teenager now and continues to have challenges. G.G provided her adopted daughter with the right environment, much love, and an opportunity to help her to be the best she could be. Despite all the concerns, G.G never gave up on her. It takes a special person who is willing to give so much to the others. While her children were small, she used to work part-time as a physical therapist. As her kids grew up, she decided to change her profession and applied to a physician assistant (P.A.) program. P.A. programs are intense and have a very grueling schedule. She graduated in her early 50s and continued to practice today. Her exemplary life had shown me the dignity of living quietly with the determination and the strength while abiding by the same values she exhibited when she decided not to pursue the legal action against me. Beyond that, she showed me her humanity by adopting a foster child, by walking the walk, rather than just talking the talk.

Most of my patients were very engaged in making the decisions regarding their pregnancy and the childbirth. During their first visit, I spent long-time counseling the patient about the optimal nutrition and the lifestyle for the best outcomes during the pregnancy. I also discussed with them what were considered to be signs of a healthy pregnancy or an abnormal pregnancy, and the tests required during the different stages of prenatal care. In the 1980s, new tests had been developed to screen the neural tube defects. Ultrasound technology was improving significantly and had become a part of routine testing for the evaluation of congenital malformations and accurate dating of the gestation.

Many tests done in the pregnancy were routine, but few specialized ones were performed only with the informed consent. One of the tests was Alfa Fetoprotein (AFP) to screen for the neural tube defects in the fetus. If the AFP was abnormal, the patient needed further testing with amniocentesis to confirm the diagnosis, and to enable the parents to make the emotional decision whether to carry the pregnancy or to have an abortion. I had never seen a parent who did not struggle with making such a gut-wrenching emotional choice. Some parents, who believed every child deserved life, declined these tests and decided to have the baby, no matter what the outcomes would be.

E.B's Story: Assigning Blame, a Response to an Abnormal Baby

One of my patients, E.B, came to see me for care during her second pregnancy. During her visit, I discussed with her the different tests that we could offer to screen for some congenital anomalies. One of the tests was AFP. I told her, if the results were abnormal, she would need further testing, including amniocentesis to determine if the baby indeed had neural tube defects involving the brain and spinal cord. I also discussed with her about having a routine ultrasound at 18 weeks of pregnancy. Around 16 weeks of pregnancy, I offered her the AFP test, along with the written informed consent, explaining the benefits, the risks, and the limitations of the analysis. E.B signed the informed consent declining the AFP, cosigned by my medical assistant, as a witness.

At about 18 weeks of pregnancy, she did have an ultrasound in a center that had been referred to her by her primary-care physician. In the late 1980's, to control costs, HMOs became a feature of mainstream medical practice.

Primary-care physicians were the captain of the ship and were pushed to lower the cost of healthcare. The insurance reimbursement was mostly cost based without much focus on the quality of care. Due to her HMO (health maintenance organization) insurance restriction, she had the ultrasound in a site recommended by her primary care physician. I had no control over where she could have had an ultrasound, and I was not familiar with the quality of the image. E.B's ultrasound showed her baby to be normal. Around 33 weeks, she felt that the baby was moving less. As a part of the evaluation, we performed a fetal monitoring test and another ultrasound.

The repeat ultrasound showed the baby to have a diagnosis of spina bifida, a defect in the spine, which meant the baby might have permanent paralysis of the lower extremities. It was unexpected considering the earlier ultrasound result at 18 weeks of pregnancy was normal. Understandably, the parents were in total shock, not understanding how it could have happened when everything seemed to be normal until now. There was no easy explanation, other than that the earlier ultrasound did not show the abnormality. I tried to give support to them, validating their fears and concerns. We immediately transferred E.B to the University of Michigan after the decision was made to deliver the baby at 34 weeks of pregnancy. The delivery was followed immediately by spinal surgery on the baby to achieve the best results under the circumstances. During her follow up visit, E.B expressed her dissatisfaction with the care and was naturally very upset about the baby, asking how we could have missed this significant anomaly of the baby in utero. Not wanting to assign the blame to an already grieving mother, I told her that, even though AFP test might have helped to diagnose the abnormality, she had made the best decision she could make at the time when she declined to have the test. I could never be sure if she would have chosen to terminate or to continue the pregnancy even if she had the information earlier.

I certainly could understand her grief and anger following the loss of having the perfect baby that every mother plans. During this anger phase, some patients want to hold somebody responsible for that adverse outcome. Though I could not confirm my impression, E.B appeared angry at herself for declining the AFP test that I had offered during the early pregnancy. She was carrying the heavy burden of conflicted feelings: feelings for her baby, who was alive and for whom she would be caring for and expected to love, and the guilt of wanting to have had the option of terminating the pregnancy.

She hired a lawyer and considered the possibility of a lawsuit. My care, however, had been appropriate and added documentation of her signature on the informed consent declining the AFP test confirmed it. The lawsuit was never filed once the lawyer received E.B's records. This result could have been different if I had not had the signed informed consent. I was initially hurt and upset when I received the request for records, questioning why she was trying to blame me for her decision not to have the test. As time went on, I understood her to need to blame somebody for her grief, anger, and guilt, for this "less-than-perfect" baby. I tried to imagine what it was like for her, the emotional pain she has to endure in raising a baby with such physical challenges and, even worse, to be a helpless witness to the burden her baby has to bear, growing up with the physical limitations.

My patients, like T.T; N.G; and G.G; when faced with the challenges, showed me the meaning of grace under pressure, strength, and hope. I hope I learned from their example to have more empathy for my patients' grief and anger; for the loss of their dreams of having a perfect child; whether due to the birth of a premature baby, fetal malformation, fetal death, or any other unexpected outcome.

K.M's Story: An Unwavering Faith

Most women have faith in God, whether they are church goers or not. It was humbling when I encountered the patients who, even during the profound events, such as the loss of a baby never questioned their faith in God, while enduring the grief of such a loss. Another of my patients, K.M was a healthy young woman who came in for routine pregnancy care. Around 18 weeks of gestation, when K.M had the routine ultrasound, we realized the baby had an abnormality, anencephaly with the absence of a skullcap and a small exposed brain, which is incompatible with life. It was a devastating experience, to deliver this unfathomable news to these parents who were so excited to see their baby's ultrasound pictures and were anticipating to learn the sex of their baby. There is no easy way to inform the parents, except to be empathetic and honest during the presentation, giving them the support, they need and the time to absorb the information.

I do not think I can adequately describe the emotional impact this mind-numbing, devastating news appeared to have on K.M and her husband. After listening to me describe the condition of their baby, a situation incompatible with life, these parents showed an unwavering faith in God. They decided to continue the pregnancy until K.M went into labor unless the baby died in utero.

K.M continued to come to see me for prenatal care and to listen to the fetal heart tones. One of the side effects of this type of malformation is the production of a significant amount of amniotic fluid, which resulted in making her uterus measure larger for the gestation. She was calm and never complained. I could not imagine what she was going through emotionally as she felt the baby moving, listened to the heartbeat, and as she, herself, had a more prominent tummy, as the baby grew. My conversations with her were mostly supportive in nature. She and her husband's faith in God were so strong, and their decision to allow this baby's life to continue no matter how short-lived it might be was never in doubt. I had nothing but respect and admiration for these parents, who had decided to let the pregnancy take its natural course, even knowing what the outcome would be.

At around 36 weeks, she went into labor and delivered the baby. The baby died twenty-four hours later. The parents held the baby and appropriately mourned their loss and then had a proper burial for their baby. However, they never wavered in their belief and the faith, that their baby was with God and was in a better place.

I had met many people who believe in God, but very few who, in their enormous grief, would be able to move forward without questioning God's role and fairness. Even people of deep faith, when faced with the challenges in life, often question and test their belief in the Almighty with anger, despair, and even a loss of confidence, albeit in most cases, temporarily. Very few who would not ask that if God existed, why would he allow their baby to die. It is very understandable to question God during such periods of grief and anger. I was wholly humbled by parents, like K.M and her husband, who had an absolute unwavering faith in God and accepted His will by believing that God knows better. I learned that, while their grief is no less profound than that of the other parents, their faith was absolute and involved asking no questions. It was an inspiring experience and a privilege to witness how these parents and others led their lives cherishing joys and accepting losses or failures, with the belief that God has higher plans beyond the reach of any human explanation.

Y.Y and W.W's Stories of Pregnancy: Same Cancer, Different Outcomes

Most pregnancies are uneventful for both the mothers and the babies. Most women are young and tend to have less comorbid conditions. The most common conditions affecting pregnancy are vascular disease, like hypertension or pre-eclampsia, a metabolic disease like diabetes, and other conditions, such as prematurity. Cancer in pregnancy is extremely rare. Any cancer diagnosis, by itself, has a frightening and emotional impact on the patient and her family. When a pregnant patient is diagnosed with cancer, fear is compounded, with the worries for both the mother and the baby. Many reasons contribute to the delays in the detection of malignancy during the pregnancy, such as the patient not fitting the typical age group, and the complex nature of the physiologic changes of pregnancy.

Furthermore, the Cancer treatment in a pregnant woman is complicated by the gestation of pregnancy, treatment choices, the timing of the diagnosis and the therapy, and the emotions involved in the decision-making. The benefits and the risks of treating or not treating cancer and its potential impact on the life of the mother and the baby or both are given paramount importance during this process. Learning that one of your loved ones has cancer during pregnancy is one of the most devastating experiences that families go through. Physicians who witness these experiences as they walk their patients through this frightening diagnosis are left with an emotional imprint that is difficult to forget. Around 1991, I diagnosed two pregnant patients both with the same unusual cancer, mediastinal lymphoma, each of which resulted in different outcomes for the mothers and babies.

Y.Y, a nurse by profession, came to me for her pregnancy care. During a routine prenatal visit at 12 to 14 weeks of pregnancy, she mentioned that she had felt a little lump at the base of her neck while she was consuming food or drink. During my examination, I felt a small nodule at the sternal notch while she was swallowing. She had no other symptoms. I was not sure what it was, but I thought it might be a nodule from her thyroid gland, which is an unusual area, but not unheard of, for such a growth. I referred Y.Y to a group of endocrinologists who specialize in abnormalities of the thyroid gland. She went to see one of the physicians, and after his evaluation, he tried to do a needle biopsy of the nodule which he was only able to feel when she swallowed. The location of this tumor made it impossible for him to do the biopsy. To get a diagnosis, the physician ordered a CT scan of the chest. She decided not to have the test, due to her concern for the baby's exposure to radiation during the scan.

A couple of weeks after her visit with the endocrinologist, she came to see me. I was sitting down on a stool, and she was sitting on the table. I discussed with her the importance of having the CT scan. She stated her concerns regarding the possible adverse effects from the radiation exposure on the baby and preferred to be followed by an Ear, Nose, and Throat (ENT) specialist at the hospital where she was working. In fact, she had already seen him, and he had agreed to monitor her closely. I was sympathetic to her concerns and understood her to need to protect her baby. However, during this conversation, I was looking at her neck and noticed the veins in her neck appeared more prominent on her right side. She mentioned she had seen the same thing. At that point, I insisted on her having a CT scan and made arrangements for her to have the test that very day. She did go for the test that day but decided not to consent to a contrast medium to decrease the exposure to radiation. Immediately after the scan, the radiologist called to tell me they suspected a massive tumor in her chest in the area called mediastinum, but the study result was limited because of the lack of contrast.

I called the chief of thoracic surgery at the University of Michigan and made an appointment for her to see him, in one week. By the time she went to see the physician at the University of Michigan (U of M), she had received the diagnosis of a full-blown superior vena cava syndrome as a result of the compression of the large veins in the chest from a cancerous tumor of lymph nodes, mediastinal lymphoma. Everything was happening very fast. The only path for Y.Y's survival was to terminate the pregnancy, followed by radiation and chemotherapy. I was not present at her bedside while Y.Y was facing these life-and-death decisions for herself and her baby. It must be devastating for Y.Y, to decide to terminate the pregnancy to save her own life. I felt I had abandoned her for not being at her side to hold her hand while she was going through this horrific experience. After Y.Y completed the treatment for cancer, she followed up with the physicians at U of M. I only saw her once at which time she was in remission but did not see her after that and did not know whether she ultimately survived the mediastinal lymphoma.

When I retired, another one of my patients, S.S., sent me a card wishing me the best in retirement. In that card, she also thanked me for our journey together for more than 30 years including her childbirth experiences and the diagnosis of her early breast cancer. Then to my surprise, she mentioned how grateful she was for my prompt action that led to her friend Y.Y's survival from cancer. S.S. said that Y.Y had moved to North Carolina where she was happily (still) living. All these years I had known S.S., she had never mentioned that Y.Y was her best friend. I was genuinely thankful to S.S. for giving me the update on Y.Y and the news she was leading a happy life touched me deeply.

W.W was another patient whom I never could forget. In the early phase of pregnancy, she called to say she had a mild cough, and I recommended over-the-counter cough medicine. It is not unusual for pregnant patients to have a post-nasal drip due to increased swelling of the mucous membranes. Around 32 weeks of pregnancy, I admitted her to the hospital for evaluation of pre-term labor. Her physical exam including lungs was normal.

At 36 weeks of pregnancy, she complained of shortness of breath, and her physical exam revealed a decrease in her breath sounds. A chest X-ray showed the changes in her chest suggestive either of pneumonia or a tumor. Further testing with a CT scan revealed a large mediastinal tumor, most likely lymphoma. During the two days of work-up, W.W started showing signs of the superior vena cava syndrome. It would be too presumptuous of me to say that I thoroughly understood what W.W, her husband, and their family were going through when they heard the diagnosis of cancer. It turned their world upside down, changing their normal expectations from an anticipated birth, still one month away, to a life-threatening diagnosis of cancer.

Many patients are eerily calm at the initial shock of hearing such a diagnosis, with their thoughts and emotions spinning out of control, it is hard for them to understand anything we discuss afterward. We did not have too much time. I held W.W's hand while I explained her diagnosis and the plans ahead. Touch and hugs give more comfort than we understand. There was not much time to consider all that she might have to go through, but we discussed the immediate steps. I focused on what the immediate next action was, which was to deliver the baby. I delivered a healthy baby boy by cesarean section. The plan after that was to transfer her and the baby to the U of M Hospital for her to receive immediate chemotherapy.

How could I know or describe the conflict of emotions, between the joy of celebrating the birth of their newborn, while thinking about the concerns and challenges that lay ahead for this newborn's mother? As a physician, I could empathize and offer the support, the love, and the hope to W.W, but it would be an overstatement if I said I was able to walk in her shoes and understand the fear, the anxiety, and the hope that such a patient feels.

I was and am still in disbelief, that in a short period, I had two patients W.W and Y.Y, with a diagnosis of this rare cancer in pregnancy, mediastinal lymphoma. Every cancer diagnosis is a journey, riddled with hope, fear, anxiety, and acceptance. One's ability to surrender to the uncertainty of life and find the joy of living as a gift perhaps helps a person to move forward, whether one outlives cancer or not. Most importantly, I wanted to give her hope. I remember my conversations with W.W, including her asking me if she would survive the cancer. I gave her reassurance that it was possible and that the only other patient I had ever encountered with the same diagnosis, Y.Y, had successfully gone into remission. That reassurance was the best I could give at that moment in time. However, my hopeful prediction did not come true. I learned her disease was in an advanced stage and had already spread to distant organs. It gave me great sadness to hear that she did not survive her cancer. I often thought about how much she must have struggled to survive, the emotional and physical pain and suffering she must have gone through, helplessly succumbing to this devastating cancer. It was difficult to imagine what she felt, knowing that every day she lived was a reminder to her that she would never see her two little children grow up and that they would grow up without knowing their mother.

Two pregnant mothers with the same diagnosis had entirely different outcomes: Y.Y survived but lost her baby to survive cancer; W.W did not survive cancer, but her baby did! I struggled with trying to make sense of the difference in outcomes in my two patients with the same diagnosis, why one patient had such a delay in manifesting the signs of the superior vena cava syndrome. What could I have done differently? Within just a few years, I had had two pregnant patients with a very rare non-

Hodgkins mediastinal lymphoma, which has an incidence of 0.8 in 100,000 patients. I wondered if I should perform tests in every patient who has a mild cough with a post-nasal drip, given the increased mucus production and swelling of mucous membranes in pregnancy.

It is normal to question and wonder if there was anything I could have done differently. As we have learned more about cancers, we know not all malignancies with the same diagnosis behave the same, progress the same, or result in the same prognosis. We have learned the prognosis depends not just on the stage, but also on the genetic makeup of the tumor, and the grading of the tumor cells that cause some tumors to grow and spread faster than others.

In spite of what I do understand, as a physician, I was always burdened with the thought of what I could have done differently to save W.W's life. I do not have any answers, yet I am bothered by the idea that I could not change this mother's outcome. Whenever I think about W.W, my heart always hurts for her children who had to grow up without their mother's love.

As a physician, I felt helpless during encounters with those of my patients who experienced the most devastating challenges, whether it was a complicated childbirth, an abnormality of the baby, an anomaly incompatible with life, the loss of a baby or a mother affected by cancer. Every one of these experiences left lifelong impressions, which left an emotional scar by my inability to change the outcomes, to heal them and make them whole. At the same time, it made me understand my limitations as a human. I knew my patients felt helpless with no ability to control their destiny.

Personal Stories

During these years, my husband and I learned we would not be able to have children. After much discussion, we decided not to adopt any children, and we made peace with our decision. Each of us, being in a medical specialty that involves babies was a real irony in our life. There is the saying that God has his plans, and we have ours, but ours do not count. I honestly believed that God had a purpose for my life and being a mother was not one of them. My patients never judged me or ever said that my lack of experience as a parent should prevent me from advising them. My husband and I are not the ones who looked back, and we chose to move forward in life.

In June of 1981, my parents came to the U.S. for the first time to visit me. It had been a long time since I had seen my parents, which was when I went to India in October of 1977. During these three and a half years, I had been unable to visit them due to the responsibilities of starting a new solo practice and being on daily call. My parents had not been able to come to see me because my mother had been the caregiver to my maternal grandmother, who was in her late 80s and who lived in our home. In 1980, my grandmother died at the age of 91. It took my parents another year to get their affairs in order and to obtain their passports and tourist visas.

My Father's Story: A Journey of Dementia and My Understanding of Dying

My parents were delighted to see me, but I noticed some changes in my father, changes which I was not sure were due to the change in culture or to the language barrier. My father had been a "people person," a leader in the community, and the person who never backed down from any challenge. I was not sure how to explain the change. My mother, on the other hand, adjusted very well and cooked some of my favorite Indian dishes, which were ready to eat when I came home tired. Most of us, no matter what our background is, tend to go into the denial when facing the problems that involve a family member. My parents were pleased to see how happy I was in my personal and professional life in my new home. They got to know my husband better. That was the most extended period we had spent together since I was married.

I took them on a trip to Washington D.C., to visit the Washington Monument, the Lincoln and Jefferson Memorials and the White House, the pillars of democracy. My father, who had been so actively engaged in politics for most of his life, was very subdued. On the other hand, my mother, who always had enjoyed the history, loved it.

Though I was unable to figure out my father's lack of interest in our trip to Washington, still I was not too worried about him or his health. After all, his parents had led very active lives and were well into their mid-80s before they died. He was one of eight children, and all of them were very healthy, both mentally and physically.

My father wanted to go home to India after only a couple of months, even though their visas were for six months. I just thought that he was bored, sitting at home while my husband and I were working long hours to meet the demands of our busy schedules. My parents went home after staying with me for just a couple of months.

From that time on, I made sure we saw each other at least every couple of years. Meanwhile, I thought my parents would be happier if they lived closer to my sisters, one of whom lived in Hyderabad, our state capital. I thought my father would be able to lead an active life being closer to the place where the political decisions were made. I also thought they would be happier being closer to their two grandsons. My younger sister lived in Chennai, the capital of Tamilnadu, and had two daughters. My parents could go to visit them every few months and enjoy spending time with them, too, or so I thought. I went to visit them in 1983 and realized that none of these changes had brought any improvements in my father's demeanor, and he had become even more withdrawn.

My husband and I moved to a new home in 1984. In 1985, I wanted my parents to come to visit me. While they were here, I finally understood that my father was going through mental changes. Concerned, I ordered a CT scan of his brain. The CT scan confirmed what I was afraid of, and showed atrophic changes in his brain, suggestive of dementia. We had to watch his every move. He was only 65 years old, and I suspect he had had early changes from dementia beginning in his late 50s. My mother and my sisters gave him the best care that was humanly possible.

Although I felt guilty because of my inability to provide support to my mother and sisters, who had enormous caregiving responsibilities, I was comforted knowing he was receiving the best care available. Whenever I went to see him, I could see further deterioration, with fewer lucid moments.

I looked at my father as two different people. This man with dementia was not the same person whom I had known as my father when I was growing up. It was like the network of wires in the brain were snapped. What triggered them to disconnect? Every family goes through this conflict when a family member has dementia. Even as a physician, I could not get my arms around the causes of these significant changes in his brain. I had many unanswered questions. Neither his parents nor any of his siblings had had dementia. What made my father so vulnerable to dementia at such an early age is still an enigma to me today. No matter what the causes were, the human toll this disease had taken on family members is indescribable.

In 1988, my parents and my niece and nephew visited me in the States. My sisters did not support the idea of them coming here for a visit. When I saw my father, I understood why. He had deteriorated significantly. He exhibited the signs and symptoms of dementia with a Parkinsonian component with frequent falls, stiffness in his body, loud screams, and talking during sleep. The only blessing during his entire disease process was he never ceased to recognize people. During one of his lucid moments, my father told my nephew and my niece the story of how I had come to the U.S. with very little money in my pocket and, nonetheless, had made it. Since I had moved here and during our previous visits, he had never mentioned anything specific about me being successful in my new country. I could see the pride in his eyes. I will cherish that moment and always remember the image I hold of my father sitting on my deck, talking to my nephew and niece about his daughter, and being proud. That was a gift I would never have had if he had not come to visit me.

Six months after the visit, in January 1989, my father became very ill and was hospitalized for a brief time. At this time, he was semi-conscious, and we decided to bring him home to die. My husband and I went to visit my father to say good-bye. Amidst my profound sadness, I learned so much about life, not in my role as a physician, but as a person. As a physician, I was having difficulty watching him die. I started intravenous fluids, so he would not be dehydrated, monitoring his blood pressure and urine output constantly. My instincts as a physician took over, and I felt as if I needed to do more to save him from dying. My mother, the wise woman, in spite of her anticipated loss, asked me what the purpose was of administering intravenous fluids and inserting a Foley catheter. With her help, I came to realize I was not making him any better, but I was prolonging his suffering. It dawned on me it was time for me to fully step into the role of being a daughter of my dying father, instead of serving as his physician.

I immediately removed the I.V. line. My older sister arranged a person who would give him baths daily. All my father's brothers, sisters, nephews, and nieces visited him frequently. He was surrounded by all his family, who genuinely cared for him and loved him. At one of those visits, he opened his eyes, looked around at everyone, and was able to recognize each person by name. It made me feel spiritually whole, knowing that he knew my husband and I were there, too. During the remaining days of his life, the family was able to feed him small sips of liquids.

After two weeks, I had to leave my dying father to return to my busy practice, knowing Dr. Maicki had been covering for me for two weeks without a break and was due to go on a once-a-year vacation with his wife. Though my family never judged me for leaving my dying father's bedside, I felt overwhelming guilt at the thought of leaving my sick father. I never stopped having the regret of abandoning my mother and the family when I should have been with them. However, that was the price I had to pay for trying to balance between my family and my duty. I fed my father with sacred water, kissed him, and said my goodbyes. I hugged my mother, with an emotion hard for me to describe, and gave her words of comfort, knowing what was to come. I talked to her about how my father would be at peace and in a better place with no more suffering. My conversations with my mother also allowed me to comfort myself and accept my father's impending death. I still carry that image of my mother standing on the balcony, waving goodbye to me.

When I arrived home in the States, my brother-in-law called to inform me that my father had died during my long journey. The date was Feb. 4th, 1989. It took me more than a year to recover from my father's loss. Anyone who goes through grief understands that one does not feel the emotion every minute of every day. I would be overcome with the grief unexpectedly. Sometimes while I was driving alone, I would find myself crying uncontrollably. I spent much time talking to my sisters and my mother, finding solace in our shared experiences. These conversations helped me to recover and make peace with myself for not being there.

I did not understand until afterward how much I had learned from my father's death. Recollecting those two weeks, I remember how beautiful it had been to see my father surrounded by his immediate and extended family, celebrating his life, telling stories about him, laughing and crying at the same time. He had looked peaceful and comfortable without the interventions or disruptions, which would have happened if he had been in the hospital. It gave me great comfort knowing we had made the right decision, to bring him home from the hospital and that he had died peacefully at home, surrounded by his loving family. In later years, I used to say my father had the best death any human being could ever have. I have great memories, whenever I think of my father's death, not regarding losing him, but regarding how he was allowed to die.

I had read Elizabeth Kubler- Ross's *Death and Dying* and intellectually understood the stages of grief: denial, anger, bargaining, depression, and acceptance. As I went through all the stages of grief, I came to a better understanding of the meaning of life and death, influenced by a sense of spirituality in life and dignity in death. Every personal experience can be the seed for a life lesson. Coming to realize my father's dementia, seeing his diminishing brain through the marvels of medical technology, and witnessing his vulnerabilities gave me a new perspective. I gained an empathy through which I could relate to another's loss and grief at a more spiritual level. My personal experience reemphasized my belief that we are all bonded by these shared human experiences as one family on this planet we call earth, despite our perceived visible differences in culture and ethnicity.

My father was a very fortunate man, able to die peacefully at home, surrounded by love, laughter, and conversations celebrating his life. However, many families are reluctant to have the necessary discussions about the death and dying, talks that might allow a more desirable end. After my experience with my father's death, I became a great proponent of advanced medical directives and now believe everyone should make their dying wishes known so that those wishes may come true.

As physicians, we often fall short of helping patients in planning advanced medical directives before they become ill. Most people do not think about or want to face the naked truth that we are born to die, and not all diseases are curable. Physicians who are trained to save lives are not well trained in how to counsel families when continuing the treatment becomes a continuation of the suffering of their loved one. The family, often in their grief, is least likely to be able to make such a difficult decision when their loved one is suffering from illness with no hope of recovery. Also, the family members often do not agree with each other, in deciding what the best treatment for their loved one is. Advanced medical directives, which give an understanding of the patient's wishes, can work as a guide for the family and the physicians in these most emotionally charged circumstances. When the treatment becomes futile, these directives may help a family carry out their family member's wishes to allow them to die in peace without intervention and the suffering, from the tubes sticking out from every part of his or her body.

Another aspect of healthcare that we continue to struggle with is our inadequate system of communication between members of the healthcare team and the patients. In the book *Heart Sounds,* by Martha Weinman Lear, a New York Times reporter, described the challenges she faced after her husband, a urologist, suffered a heart attack. She explained how she and her husband were disappointed with the lack of communication from his physicians and the mistakes that were made along the way by the hospital, interns, and residents. She correctly described the bureaucracy in healthcare systems that I recognized and to which I could relate. She talked about the pain and the suffering, the love and loss the patient and the family had to endure in witnessing their loved one's health decline every day.

Her book was truly inspirational to me in examining the multiple facets of the health care system. Our primary responsibility first and foremost is to the patient and the family. How do we address their needs and concerns? How do we learn to walk in their shoes and discuss the actual status of the patient's condition, while allowing time for them to process and grieve such a significant change in their life? How do we make sure the entire healthcare team—attending physicians, interns, residents, and nurses—is on the same page regarding patient care? How do we train our interns and residents that each patient is a *person*, not a *condition* and that the healthcare provider's solemn responsibility is to listen to the patient's concerns even when they are tired at the end of a long shift? What a physician may think of as being a trivial issue may not be insignificant to the patient. How do we make sure the patients and their families can engage and participate in the patient's health care? How can the physician help the patient and his/her family to become an advocate for the management of the patient's health care?

At the end of her book, Weinman Lear poignantly states her disappointments in the health care provided for her husband, particularly the suffering he had to endure and the health care team's lack of communication, right up until he died. She understood, how the physicians could have made the mistakes that are human, in the management of her husband with a chronic condition over four years. What bothered her the most was the physicians' lack of empathy and the recognition of the mistakes they made. When a family member is suffering from any chronic illness, we, as physicians, fail to recognize and acknowledge the family's grief, for their and our inability to make their loved one better. Finally, what she struggled with and grieved for was the realization that no one could make the impossible possible, no one could make him well again, make him whole the way he was before his heart attack.

A Time of Transition for My Department

In 1988, Dr. Krohn, our department chair, decided to move on. Just before he left, he shared with me that I was the busiest obstetrician in the department, a surprise to both him and me. We went out for lunch before his retirement, and I thanked him for his role in helping me achieve my goal of becoming an obstetrician and gynecologist. He encouraged me to get involved in the expanding field of gynecology, including minimally invasive surgery.

In 1988, Dr. Roger Hertz from Ohio's Case Western University, an intellect and a specialist in maternal and fetal medicine with many publications under his belt, became our new chairman of the department. He is smart and intense, cared deeply about the department and decided to develop a new faculty, and enhance the engagement of attending physicians in the resident education. Roger reached out to the leaders in the department to discuss his plans. He was planning to begin morning resident educational rounds and asked me to participate one morning every week. During the morning rounds, the residents were asked to present all patients in labor and delivery and gynecology service, discussing the status of the patients and their treatment plans.

These rounds helped to provide a successful transition of care between the outgoing on-call residents and the incoming residents during the day shift. This practice of having morning rounds resulted in lively discussions about the pathophysiology of individual patient conditions, their treatment plans, and the decision process. Everyone learned from it, including the attending physicians. I participated in weekly rounds for eleven years until I stopped practicing obstetrics. The morning rounds continued even after Roger Hertz retired and still is part of the department's residency education program. The transition of patient care rounds during shift changes are not only educational, but they have been shown to contribute to the improved patients' care, safety, and outcomes.

Dr. Roger Hertz retired in 1992. We developed a strong friendship during the four years of his tenure as the department chair. His wife, Dawn, became one of my good friends. That friendship continues to date. They live in

Florida during the winter, and we get together with them a couple of times during their visit to Michigan each year.

From 1985-1991, Dr. Maicki and I continued to manage our busy practice with a schedule of 36 hours on and 12 hours off. The two of us were performing about 20% of all the deliveries at Providence Hospital. Though having had the privilege of delivering babies was a very satisfying shared experience with our patients, the hectic schedule came with a tremendous personal sacrifice to our spouses. So, in 1991, another well-respected physician, Dr. Anthony Boutt, who also had a busy practice, expressed his desire to share night call with us, and we gladly agreed to the arrangement.

Women's Health: Teenage Years to Menopause

[A] woman is like a tea bag—you never know how strong she is until she gets in hot water.

--- Eleanor Roosevelt

The practice of gynecology focuses on women's health from adolescence through the remainder of a woman's life. During both the pre-adolescence and menopausal transitions in life, girls and women experience significant physical, hormonal, and emotional changes. These changes start with the onset of the menses and cyclical hormonal changes and involve an understanding of sexuality and the responsibility that comes with it. At about age ten; many girls experience the prepubertal changes of the breast and female hair growth pattern, which is very confusing for many girls and for some, it can be scary.

In the past generations, mothers usually did not discuss or explain to their daughters about the ensuing changes during adolescence and teenage years, which could have been an overwhelming experience for an adolescent. Fortunately, nowadays, the majority of the mothers and schools teach children about what to expect and discuss the physiology of the body, to help them to cope with, both the physical and emotional changes that come with the surging hormones. It is an understatement to say that the teenage years are the most difficult for both the parents, especially for the mothers and their adolescent daughters. Mothers tend to be more engaged in their children's day-to-day welfare and worry about their children getting into harmful activities like alcohol, drugs and engaging in sex too early, especially unprotected sex. While mothers are trying to prevent their teenage daughters from making any mistakes, the daughters feel they are all grown up, and they think they are fully capable of figuring out what is right and what is wrong and don't need to be supervised as children.

Fortunately, most teenagers come out of their teenage years safely and move on to have a healthy life, having learned from their mistakes. Such is the cycle of life. My advice to mothers was to give some space to their daughters by ignoring rainbow hair colors or body piercing and focusing more on how to avoid the situations involving drugs, alcohol, and unprotected sex.

Some mothers felt by just having a conversation about contraception and the importance of using condoms to prevent sexually transmitted diseases, they would be giving their daughters a sign of approval, for them to engage in sexual activity. I also saw mothers who had an honest conversation with their daughters regarding their concerns and the consequences of specific behaviors during the teenage years. At the same time, mothers were open to listening to their daughter's need for contraception, even though they did not agree with the teenager's decision to engage in sexual activity. These mothers understood, their daughters would be better off if they received STD and contraceptive counseling from a physician. If necessary, they were okay with the contraception prescription to prevent teenage pregnancy. Unfortunately, many times, my adolescent patients who were using contraception did not want to talk to their mothers. Conversations build trust, and I believe are the stepping-stones for long-term relationships. It had been my observation that every generation tends to resist behaving like the generation before them or taking their advice. However, it brought a smile to my face when I observed daughters emulate their mothers, and the mothers behave more like their mothers, which they swore they would never be during the moments of frustration!

As a woman moves on from her teenage years and becomes a young woman, she becomes busy trying to figure out her future, through her relationships and career moves. Trying to balance between a career and a relationship can be challenging. When a woman settles down in a relationship, married or otherwise, she starts planning the next phase in her life; that is to start a family. Motherhood is a significant change in woman's life which involves many adjustments and adaptations. It truly represents a new life. Most women are working mothers, trying to balance their forever demanding careers and the expectations of being a mother could be challenging. There are some tradeoffs of being a working mother, such as being late to or missing work on one hand and missing dinners with their children and events at school on the other hand. Though many fathers share the responsibility of caring for their children, most mothers feel more responsible for the care and nurture of her children. It could be because of the more traditional stereotypes of the family structure, or it could be related to the natural nurturing encoded in the woman's biology. This emotional conflict between the roles of motherhood and career can create a feeling of inadequacy which casts long shadows for the rest of their lives.

For two to three decades in their life, women, working or at home mom, are pre-occupied with, being a mother, and busy caring for their family with care, love, and dedication. Once all the children leave the house, they go through the mixed emotions of joy and sadness. Mothers are happy that the children are moving on with their lives as expected, while at the same time, feeling lost by not having the day-to-day interactions with them. An empty nest may create a vacuum in a woman's life, which may lead to anxiety and depression. Also, a mother's concerns for her child in college without supervision may be overpowering and paralyzing. A mother always worries about her children, no matter how old they are, whether she is in her forties and concerned about her children in college, or in her eighties, worrying about their children going through the mid-life crisis. As children grow and become young adults, as they spread their wings and take off into life, many mothers feel lost and emotionally vulnerable.

E.E's Story: The Process of Letting Go

One of my patients, E.E, had one child, a daughter, A.E, who went to college in Miami, Florida. E.E felt lost and missed her daughter very much. They had been very close, and she missed being near her and missed hearing her voice daily. Learning of this, A.E promised her mother she would call her every day. As a result, E.E never left home for any event the entire first year of her daughter's college so that she would not miss A.E's call and the joy of listening to her voice. She was paralyzed and was unable to move on with her own life. During a casual conversation at a routine visit, E.E confided how much she missed her daughter and what she had been doing—or not doing—for the last year. She was very happy for her daughter for attending the college of her choice, but E.E did not have the tools to cope with this significant change in her life. We discussed the pressure and guilt her daughter A.E could be going through, knowing her mother was waiting for her call and for deciding to move to a state far away from home.

We talked about how important it was that she moved on with her life and that she needed to realize that she could return A.E's call afterward. It was not that she did not know this simple fact; but, someone needed to reinforce that it did not diminish her love for her daughter if she did not pick up the phone the minute A.E called. We also talked about how it would decrease the burden of guilt A.E would feel if she missed making the call one night.

I was pleasantly surprised, during her next visit when she told me how much our conversation had helped her to move on to the next phase of her life. When A.E graduated, she decided to move to California, and E.E and her husband helped her move and gave her all the support A.E needed. E.E continued to update me about her joyful visits to

California. After a few years in California, A.E decided to move back home to Michigan. That was great news for me to hear, and I felt I had played a small role in redirecting E.E's life. Seeing E.E adapting to the changes in her life was just one example of a mother's ability to adjust to a long-distance relationship with her daughter. It ultimately helped to forge the strong bonds that pulled A.E back to Michigan, despite the years of separation.

Menopause: Symptoms, Treatment, and Controversy

Just about the time her children are leaving home, a woman faces another major transition in her life. Women during the peri-menopause and menopause, experience declining hormonal production and the cessation of menstrual periods, ending her reproductive years. Menopause is a normal physiologic event, but symptoms of menopause sometimes can be disabling. There is nothing ordinary about these symptoms for a woman who is going through it.

During the perimenopausal period, with its irregular production and declining levels of hormones, women go through varying degrees of symptoms that may be confusing and sometimes scary. Many women wonder if something is wrong with them. During the perimenopausal and menopausal years, women may experience irregular periods: frequent or less frequent, short or prolonged, heavy or scant. Many women also experience one or more symptoms, including hot flashes, decreased libido, painful sex, sometimes mood changes, and occasionally even nausea and dizziness, which has a significant impact on their daily life. Any or all such changes might cause additional insecurity for women who were already emotionally charged and affected by empty nest syndrome after their children had left home. Frequent periods or prolonged bleeding should be further evaluated to rule out benign or malignant pathology. Sometimes abnormal thyroid function, certain breast cancer drug treatments, and in very few cases rare cancers may also lead to hot flashes, similar to those in menopause.

In the early years of my practice, it was common to treat all menopausal woman with the hormone therapy, whether the patient was symptomatic or not. Estrogen helped hot flashes and painful sex, and progesterone reduced the risk of uterine cancer. At that time, physicians did not provide much counseling about the benefits and the risks of hormone therapy. Hormone therapy was also believed to show a decrease in the incidence of osteoporosis and cardiovascular disease. This combined hormone therapy, with all its benefits, was routinely prescribed to all women.

In the 1990s, there was a significant movement toward alternative and complementary medicine, with the baby-boomer generation challenging the norms at the time. Hormone therapy received the most attention because women were going through menopause and wanted to consider the alternative treatments. In response to the women's needs, the pharmaceutical industry started a new line of plant-based hormone therapy consisting of the bioactive hormones: estradiol and hydroxyprogesterone. I prescribed this plant-based hormone therapy to all my patients. However, there was much suspicion with any pharmaceutical products. Women wanted the so-called natural products. With the increasing demand for natural hormones, local pharmacies started to compound the hormones, and many physicians who were not gynecologists became hormone doctors. It became a multibillion-dollar industry. Celebrities got into it, too. Many authors published the books, some legit and some not so legit. Anything with the word "Natural" was better and made them believe it was all safe. The FDA has no regulations for most of these products, and the patients did not know if they were receiving the correct dosage of the drugs that matched the prescription. Even worse there was no way of knowing if the drugs had any contaminants or the risks associated with them.

I understood where the patients were coming from and their need to question the pharmaceutical industry, which had been shown to manipulate the studies of some drugs. Later, some of the drugs were shown to have harmful effects on many patients. This distrust was and still is rampant, and the alternative medicine industry took advantage of this anti-establishment movement, flooding the market with all kinds of supplements, including anti-aging products, and hormones labeled"Natural," with the subliminal message, implying no risk.

The sales pitch and the marketing genius of "natural" hormone therapy with its *absolute security of safety* is a tide that I was unable to overcome. My passionate discussion to convince my patients that the pharmaceutically produced plant-based hormones with a standardized drug dosage might be at least as safe as the natural hormones frustrated some of my patients and angered others. I was unable to convince them that I was not against alternatives nor did I disagree that some of these supplements had benefits, but I did want them to understand what the possible side effects could be. Unfortunately, there are no regulations to warn the public of the side effects (and occasional deadly consequences) of herbal products. I tried to emphasize, to no avail, the necessity to buy the products with adequate scientific information. Such was the marketing influence of the alternative medicine industry.

In 1999, when I stopped practicing obstetrics, I realized the need to start a comprehensive center for the menopause and women's health. I wrote a proposal and presented it to the hospital administration, explaining the need for and the importance of creating a resource center, which could help women during the menopause with a holistic approach. I hoped this center would address the healthy lifestyle, stress reduction, and biofeedback which could help to alleviate the symptoms of menopause, reduce the risks of cardiovascular disease, and osteoporosis, all conditions that may afflict women after menopause. I also wanted this to be a good resource center for women, to learn about the benefits and the risks of hormones, and herbal products. After a few years of discussion back-and-forth, I realized the administration did not share my vision, and I gave up on that idea of developing a comprehensive center for women's health and menopause.

A.A.'s Story: Menopausal Symptoms and the Mind-Body Connection

We should address the treatment of menopausal symptoms with a holistic approach. Hormone therapy in a symptomatic woman should not be the sole treatment option, but managing menopause should include lifestyle changes as well. Women can learn to identify the triggers for hot flashes, like physical and emotional stress, and intake of caffeine or alcohol, but changing the lifestyle is never easy. It does not have to be all or none. Moderation is the key. One cannot underestimate the impact that exercise has in helping to produce endorphins, which have a calming effect on anxiety and stress. In more than 80% of women, significant menopausal symptoms like hot flashes and insomnia gradually abate and become tolerable without any impact on their daily life. In symptomatic women, hormone therapy is very beneficial, along with the adoption of lifestyle changes. Hormone therapy should be reevaluated on an individual basis, and many women successfully wean off of the hormone therapy after three to five years of treatment.

Risks from hormone therapy had been shown to be less significant when a woman is in her fifties and especially in the first five years of treatment. Intravaginal estrogen therapy may be continued to alleviate dyspareunia (painful sex) that many women experience from atrophic changes caused by declining estrogen. A minority of the women have difficulty managing their menopausal symptoms without the hormone therapy and may require prolonged treatment. Some women, many years after their menopausal symptoms had abated and who were not on any hormones, used to call our office for a prescription of hormones solely because they were experiencing a new onset of hot flashes. In these situations, we need to evaluate the patients further, and the hormone therapy is unlikely to help the symptoms.

A.A. made an appointment with me to discuss her significant hot flashes and insomnia, which were affecting her daily quality of life. I had known A.A. for decades and delivered all her children. During peri-menopausal and menopausal office visits, she told me she was experiencing very minimal symptoms and did not require any treatment. Four years after the menopause, in 2009, A.A. started experiencing significant hot flashes affecting her quality of life.

During the visit, I explained to her that it was unlikely her symptoms were due to the decline in hormones. A.A. had experienced very minimal symptoms in the acute phase of menopause, which is when such symptoms tend to be most significant. Other causes of hot flashes, after a prolonged latent period of asymptomatic menopause, could be from an abnormal thyroid condition, rare medical conditions, drugs or the result of acute situational stress. Her thyroid function test results were normal. There had been no changes in her medications or the usual culprits, like alcohol or caffeine intake, or exercise habits. During the visit, we went into a "deep-dive" mode to identify the everyday stress inducing causes. The most common causes of stress usually arise from the relationships, responsibilities, medical and behavioral issues, and financial and job insecurities.

Many women feel stressed and sandwiched between the responsibilities for their own families and the care and the attention required for their older parents. We went through A.A.'s relationship with her husband and the children, which she expressed were going well. Her children were in their teenage years, but they were not manifesting any behavior issues that caused alarm. Her parents died a few years before, and she appeared to be at the right stage of her life without any unusual stresses.

As we kept peeling back the layers of onion, I asked her if there were any financial concerns. It was in 2009; the financial crisis was real, financial markets were crashing, and people were losing their jobs. As a result of the recession, many families were feeling significant insecurity about their future financial security, especially as they looked at the stock investment accounts becoming less every month. However, I learned that A.A.'s husband's job was secure, and there were no immediate concerns. During our conversation about finances, A.A. told me it was she who oversaw the couple's investment portfolio.

At that time, the minute-to-minute updates on financial cable news channels were having a significant and probably unintended "brainwashing" effect on the individuals, sending them into the rabbit hole of thinking that they might never come out of this crisis. A.A. did not realize the impact of listening to these cable channels all day. Such underlying stress produces natural chemicals in our bodies, epinephrine and norepinephrine, which in turn affects the thermal regulatory centers in the brain, causing hot flashes and insomnia.

After much discussion, I was able to convince A.A. to stop watching or listening to the financial cable news and, instead, to engage in activities that give her joy and happiness. Concerning her investment management, I advised A.A. to devote about half an hour of quiet time every day to decide what changes she needed to make in her portfolio. I asked her to make a follow-up appointment in three months after she had adopted these lifestyle changes. During her follow-up appointment, A.A. let me know how surprised she was when she was able to sleep better with minimal hot flashes once she had adopted the lifestyle changes I had suggested. She laughingly added that not only was she sleeping better, but her husband had followed her lead and was sleeping better, too.

I had noticed how the audio-visual onslaught of the messages impacted some individuals. Many women felt anxiety after watching the first Gulf War on television, and some of them requested sleeping medication. These are the perfect examples of that; we do not have to be physically sick to feel sick. Peeling the layers of human emotions to get to the core issues allows a physician to address the cause and effect, which helps the physicians to treat the patients accordingly. A constant bombardment of messages, feeding off of each other, tends to be more harmful than positive. Constant messaging can have such an impact on our brain and is another example of bio-feedback responses, either positive or negative. The mind-body-spirit, the axis of thoughts, emotions, and physical reactions should not be left on the backburner of a diagnosis but should be as important as the physical evaluation.

My Changing Practice: 1991-2003

Love and peace of mind do protect us.
They allow us to overcome the problems that life hands us.
They teach us to survive to live now,
to have the courage to confront each day.

--- Bernie Siegel

1991 to 2003 were the most transformational years in our practice and involved many changes like increasing from three to eight-member group. On the top of that, I became an employed physician in 1996, after eighteen years of private practice. I had to learn to adjust to these significant changes, which was not easy. Most OB-GYN's became employed by the hospitals to help to reduce the cost of malpractice insurance. Reimbursement is not valued equally across all the specialties. It is well known; the insurance companies pay less for the prevention of illnesses and the cognitive medicine and more for the treatments, the latest interventions or the advanced imaging. Most other specialties do not understand the complexities of care and the decision-making process in obstetrics and gynecology.

Women's health is one of the most underappreciated medical specialties as it requires complex decision-making, which often involves managing two lives, a mother, and her baby or complicated surgeries affecting women's health. Women's health appears to be weighed so differently regarding the value of care. Could it be related to how a woman's position is reflected in general society, for instance, with the acceptance of less than equal pay for same work?

Beginning in the '90s, more women postponed starting the families into their early 30's so they could establish their careers before having children. Because of the advancing maternal age, risks for hypertension, diabetes, obesity and morbid obesity, as well as pre-eclampsia, had increased. In the '90s, diagnostic capabilities of other comorbid conditions like thrombophilia (a genetic disorder that increases blood clotting) increased by the availability of new tests. We learned the increased risk posed by these conditions for both the mother and the baby. In higher-risk pregnancies, often decisions had to be made to deliver a baby early to save the mother's life. The premature labor and the deliveries posed the highest risk for newborn infants. Prematurity, despite significant advancements in neonatal care, was then, and is still, the leading cause of the infant mortality. Maternal infections, in spite of all the advances made, are one of the leading causes of morbidity/mortality to the mother and the baby.

Z.Z's Story: Different Times, Different Mindset, Different Decision

While the infectious disease has been impacting communities since the beginning of time, exposure to infections during pregnancy increases the risk of congenital anomalies. Rubella was one of the success stories, with its mass immunization program, which protected many children from being born with the congenital anomalies that would have had devastating effects. Recently the development of a hepatitis vaccination helped to decrease fetal transmission, which is not always practiced uniformly in all corners of the world. Nonetheless, pregnant women are exposed to many infections, viruses like., parvovirus, Coxsackie, HIV, Zika, for which there are no vaccinations, and which may have severe consequences for a baby. Also, infections like syphilis, a sexually transmitted disease, and Toxoplasmosis, a parasitic infection acquired from the handling of contaminated cat feces, increase the risk of congenital abnormalities when left untreated.

Many households have cats as pets. Prenatal counseling included instructing them not to clean the cat litter as it could increase the risk of toxoplasmosis in the mother, which in turn increases the risk of congenital anomalies. Some patients were unaware of this problem and were already exposed to the infection by cleaning the cat litter before starting the prenatal care.

Z.Z was one of my pregnant patients who was not aware of the risk posed by cat litter. I tested her blood for toxoplasmosis in early pregnancy, which showed very high blood IgM titers, suggesting exposure to the disease during her pregnancy. I compassionately explained to Z.Z, the risks of visual, hearing and cognitive impairment to the baby. Then I went further discussing with Z.Z the choices in front of her, either to continue the pregnancy with possible risks to the baby or not to continue. I told her that she could count on my support, no matter what her decision would be. Z.Z decided to continue the pregnancy. After consulting with the genetics department, I gave Z.Z an option to have a procedure that would test the umbilical cord blood to confirm whether the baby was infected.

The decade before Z.Z's complicated pregnancy, there was a development of new procedures to advance the fetal diagnosis in utero. At the time of Z.Z's, case, there were very few centers nationally who were performing the test called cordocentesis. One of these centers was Yale University. Z.Z was willing to travel to Connecticut and have the test done at the Yale School of Medical Science. Just within ten years after I started practice, I was a witness to this incredible pace of progress in ultrasound technology. Such advances enabled us to draw blood from the umbilical cord of the fetus in utero, to diagnose the diseases that could not be otherwise diagnosed. Cordocentesis is also used to transfuse the babies in utero with blood incompatibilities, saving the lives of many. Z.Z had a successful cordocentesis with no complications. At the time of the test, the baby had tested negative for toxoplasmosis. The specialist advised treatment with a drug pyrimethamine sulfate to prevent any future exposure of the baby to toxoplasmosis.

Pyrimethamine Sulfate was not approved by the Federal Drug Administration (FDA) to be prescribed for pregnant patients and was not available in the U.S. but was available in Canada. Special approval was obtained from the FDA, both for the prescription of the medication for the patient and to get the medication from Canada. Luckily, Detroit shares a border with

Windsor, Canada, so it was easy for the patient to get the drug. The pregnancy progressed well, we delivered a healthy baby, and the placenta was sent to be tested for toxoplasmosis to a lab in Palo Alto, California. The test was negative. During this entire ordeal, Z.Z was composed and determined to have this complicated procedure and take medications as advised to make sure her baby was healthy. It never ceased to amaze me how patients rise to the occasion during extreme situations, facing stress with such a composure that is beyond my understanding. I have seen such examples of eternal optimism and a spiritual approach that indicates a belief that the situation is in God's hands and everything is going to be all right.

Z.Z came to see me for her subsequent pregnancy, and I was baffled when she decided to terminate the pregnancy saying she was not ready to have another baby. So, her decision to continue the previous pregnancy with the complication of toxoplasmosis was not the result of a "pro-life" conviction. Could it be because she had planned the pregnancy, she was determined to have the baby, despite all the challenges she faced during the pregnancy.? Still, it was such a contradiction in how she decided to continue or terminate the pregnancy from one pregnancy to the next. By keeping the pregnancy with toxoplasmosis, she took a significant chance of having a baby with congenital anomalies, which could have led to a lifetime of dependency. Was it possible Z.Z had not known how intense the process was going to be when she decided to continue the pregnancy? Though she looked calm through the entire pregnancy and was focused on getting the tests and treatment, did she not realize the enormity of her decision? Did the next pregnancy reminded her of the burden and stress of her previous pregnancy and led to her decision to terminate the pregnancy?

Perhaps it could be simpler than that: she planned one pregnancy, and the next one she did not. I felt it was my responsibility to inform her about the risks inherent to the termination and the possible residual emotional impact she might feel unexpectedly afterward. Sometimes there may be a long road to recovery and healing. I tried to make each woman comfortable that my door was always open and gave her the option to feel free to discuss such emotions. It would be too presumptuous of me to be a moral judge of any patient, to be critical of her decision-making process and decide how the emotional responses should be unless I had been in her situation. It is an enigma of human nature. We are not always as consistent in our responses as we may expect to be. Instead, a decision may be a result of the state of mind at any given time.

In the 1990s, we started seeing more women getting pregnant in their mid-30s. The chance of a woman having a chromosomally abnormal baby increases every year but becomes statistically significant around age 35. Expectant mothers with an advanced maternal age of 35 or older, face the dilemma of making decisions whether to have the diagnostic tests for chromosomal abnormalities. Chromosomes are the carriers of our genes. The chromosomal analysis is defined as karyotyping.

Even minute changes in the chromosomes can lead to significant diseases or congenital anomalies. The majority of the chromosomally abnormal babies is the result of a random mutation that could have happened during the formation of the zygote. In the minority of babies, an inherited gene transmitted from parents is the cause of chromosomal abnormalities.

Dr.Nadler, in 1968 reported that the karyotyping of a tissue culture of amniotic fluid identified the Trisomy 21 abnormality, Down syndrome. The Down syndrome occurs when there is an extra copy of Chromosome 21, resulting in Trisomy 21. Though the most common reason for performing amniocentesis is to diagnose the chromosomal abnormalities and neural tube defects, there are hundreds of genetic disorders that can be diagnosed, from the amniotic fluid. In 1974, when I started my residency, it was the standard of practice to offer amniocentesis to women at age 35. At age 35, the risk of having a Down syndrome baby outweighs the risk of the amniocentesis procedure, such as the risk of fetal loss, rupture of amniotic membrane, and rarely, maternal infection and maternal morbidity. It is up to the parents' whether to have the test or not, after weighing the benefits, the risks. The decision to have amniocentesis was very much dependent on the personal beliefs about terminating the pregnancy or having the baby no matter what.

With the advances in technology, new tests were developed to diagnose chromosomal abnormalities earlier than 16 weeks. CVS (chorionic villus sampling) is a test of the placental tissue and can be performed in the first trimester of pregnancy to diagnose chromosomal abnormalities. This earlier stage of decision-making may have a less emotional impact on parents if they ultimately choose to terminate the pregnancy before they witness the growth of the baby and start feeling fetal movements.

Within the last decade, after the successful mapping of the human DNA, advances have been made to the degree that a simple, no-risk blood test of the mother can help screen her baby for chromosomal abnormalities, reducing the need for a potentially risky amniocentesis. Amniocentesis is advised if the blood test is inconclusive for diagnosis.

A Story of Family and Love: Down Syndrome Children

The most frequent chromosomal abnormality is Down syndrome. Some chromosomal abnormalities, like Trisomy 13 and Trisomy 18, are incompatible with life, but Down syndrome is very different. Down syndrome babies can be born with a broad spectrum of congenital anomalies from mild to significant forms of neurological deficit and cardiac defects.

In my practice, some mothers chose not to have any tests for Down syndrome, even if they were candidates, because it was not going to change their decision. Most of them had healthy babies, but some of them had babies with Down syndrome.

At birth, the Down syndrome babies have distinct facial features that a physician recognizes and, subsequently, has the uncomfortable responsibility of informing the patient of his/her suspicion and the need to perform karyotyping to confirm the diagnosis. In this situation, my approach was to sit on the bed, holding mother's hand, and say in a calm voice directly looking at the parents that I noticed mild changes in the facial features and I think we need further testing to see if the baby has Down syndrome." Then I would continue the conversation by addressing their fears and anxieties from the devastating and challenging news I just delivered. I never wanted to tell them that I was sure about the diagnosis until I received the confirmation from the test results. My approach gave the parents time to emotionally adjust to the idea of their baby having Down syndrome, a diagnosis which changes all their plans and dreams for the baby.

No matter how ready the parents think they might be to accept a baby with the Down syndrome, it does not mean they do not go through the grieving process, wondering what lays ahead for their baby. In the past, babies with Down syndrome, for the most part, were placed in the institutions. Beginning in the 1980s, many mothers fought for the assimilation of their Down syndrome children into the public-school system, augmented with the programs providing for their unique needs. Now, most of these children are adults, and some of them function at a high enough level to perform low-level jobs. One of the top performing adults with Down syndrome was actor Chris Burke.

I never heard parents of Down syndrome babies complain about the challenges of raising their children. Children with Down syndrome can be stubborn but exhibit unconditional love to everyone. Most mothers felt this unique bond of unconditional love was a blessing in their life. One of my patients expressed concern to her family about who was going to look after her son with Down syndrome after she and her husband died. She was relieved and pleased to hear that another of her sons said he would. I also had two sisters as patients, one of whom had Down syndrome, and it was a great pleasure of mine to see them together and how the older sister cared for her younger sister with Downs. The conversations between the younger sister and her older sister were so revealing of the love between them. The older sister had decided to be the guardian of her special sister when her parents got older. It was my honor and privilege, as a physician, to witness these unique relationships of unconditional love between a mother and a child or between the brothers or the sisters. Demonstrating the purest of loves in their humanity of caring for each other, I feel blessed to have had the great honor of knowing them.

V.V's Story: When One Twin Does Not Survive

With advancing maternal age and the use of fertility drugs came a higher incidence of twins or other multiple pregnancies. Multiple pregnancies increase the risks for prematurity, which is the most common cause of high infant mortality. Multiple pregnancies also have the additional complication of the babies not having equal growth, or sometimes affected by twin-to-twin transfusion increasing morbidity and mortality. In such cases, one becomes too large getting a more significant share of the blood, and the other one becomes too small not getting enough. Occasionally, such a condition can lead to the death of one twin, while the other one lives and thrives. This situation creates both an emotional and a complex-decision making process for both the mother and the physician. When one twin is doing well, and the other twin is in trouble in preterm pregnancy, it poses a moral as well as a clinical dilemma: How do you prevent harming the healthy twin while saving the life of the sick twin?

V.V, one of my patients who was carrying a twin gestation. Around 28 weeks gestation, I diagnosed her with an intrauterine fetal death of one of her twins. In V.V's case, at least the moral dilemma of saving the sick twin did not have to be taken into consideration. Now our sole focus was on how to save the living twin. As expected, to deliver the news to V.V that one of her babies had died, was difficult and challenging. It never became routine, easy or less conflicting emotionally, whenever I had to tell the mother that her baby was not alive. I was not sure how one dealt with the grieving process for the loss of one baby while worrying about the wellbeing of the other. We admitted V.V to the hospital to monitor the surviving baby with a fetal monitor and ultrasound. There was always a concern that the dead baby may produce toxins or blood clots that could lead to the death of the surviving twin in utero. V.V was patient with having to have the frequent tests to make sure her living baby was doing well. This waiting period was emotionally excruciating, involving a roller coaster of feelings not knowing the outcome, wondering and worrying if the baby will survive or not. Her mind was utterly pre-occupied with every little interruption that she had to endure during the hospitalization, that something could go wrong at any given moment and could lead to her surviving baby's death.

I could only imagine what pregnant mothers in this situation go through, away from the husband, when they are alone at night in an uncomfortable bed, unable to sleep, and worried sick about the baby. Very rarely we address these emotional issues and the psychological impact of prolonged hospitalization. As physicians, we have difficulty understanding why some mothers want to leave the hospital, even given the risk to the health of their baby. They are too scared to hear any rational argument, no matter how valid it might be.

V.V was unlike some of the mothers in this condition that I had had an interaction in my practice. Somehow, she kept her emotions in check, focusing on the living baby and taking one day at a time, patiently awaiting the 34th week of pregnancy, at which time, I planned to deliver the surviving twin. At delivery, I could not fathom her feelings of both relief and joy with the birth of her healthy baby mixed with the profound sadness for the lost baby. Every birthday of the surviving twin will be a reminder of the lost twin, and who that baby might have been if it had survived. It is an ambiguous legacy to have as the surviving twin.

I admired V.V for her poise, her calmness, her focus on the baby that was alive. She never "lost it" emotionally. I was aware that all the emotional support and counseling I tried to offer could not be enough. It was a journey that V.V had to travel alone to find some peace with what had happened. Later, during our conversations, V.V confided to me how she was able to hide the feelings of sadness, on the twins' birthday, celebrating the life and birth of one baby, while grieving the loss and death of another baby at the same time.

As a mother, she was determined and made sure that her living child was given such love and made to feel so very special so that the survivor would not have to carry the burden of her lost twin, with whom she had shared more than six months in her mother's womb. I was honored to know V.V and witness how she lived through these complex emotions and processed them to come out intact after the birth of her living child.

Prematurity: A New Scenario

Prematurity is one of the most challenging dilemmas in managing pregnancy for most obstetricians. In 1974, when I started my residency if a baby was born at 28 weeks or earlier we did not initiate any supportive treatment because the baby was unlikely to survive.

Over the years, we tried to prevent premature labor by treating pregnant women with different drugs. In the 1970s, we managed premature labor, believe it or not, with intravenous alcohol. I do not think it helped to prevent premature labor, and patients indeed became drunk, which many times resulted in uncontrollable vomiting. We later learned that, in addition to not preventing the premature labor, alcohol was dangerous for the babies in utero.

After we no longer recommended the alcohol treatment, we treated premature labor with bed rest for the mother along with many different drugs over several decades with tocolytic agents like ritodrine, terbutaline, magnesium sulfate, calcium channel blockers like Procardia and finally NSAIDS like Indocin. Controversy continues today as to whether any of these treatments help prevent premature delivery in patients who are in labor with documented cervical changes. Tocolytics may play a role in prolonging the pregnancy for at least an additional 24-

48 hours while antenatal steroids are administered to help mature the baby's lungs.

In some cases, prematurity can be dealt with before a woman goes into premature labor. A previous history of premature birth is the most significant risk factor for premature delivery. 17 hydroxyprogesterone, a hormone, which was proven to be beneficial for the prevention of premature labor is recommended for such patients, beginning at 16 weeks. Another common cause of early labor is an infection. Infections during pregnancy have been treated more aggressively with antibiotics in the last quarter century.

The most common problem for premature babies comes from their immature lungs. Immature lungs result in decreased oxygenation, which affects multiple organs and results in very high morbidity and mortality rates. Since the 1970s, significant advances were made to improve neonatal outcomes by developing drugs to help the lung maturity and oxygen-monitoring of premature babies. Neonatal intensive care units became the norm in many hospitals staffed by neonatologists, physicians who specialize in new-born illnesses.

For centuries, we have understood that some babies born extremely premature survived with no medical support. We wondered what made some survive while others did not. We explained it through the Darwinian theory of "survival of the fittest." We thought most likely the mothers of premature babies who survived had a strong genetic background and may have also had medical conditions that increased the physical stress on their body. Stress, most likely, helped to facilitate the lung maturity of the baby by increasing the production of corticosteroids, leading to better outcomes.

Prevention of premature delivery and improving the neonatal outcomes of premature babies is an evolving story. In the past three decades, with the advent of antenatal steroids and pulmonary surfactants, the survival rate of premature infants had improved even at the gestational age of as early as 23 weeks, which was unthinkable just a couple of decades earlier.

We still have many unanswered questions. What does their survival mean? How many of these babies will be intact both physically and mentally? How do we pragmatically guide pregnant mothers about the challenges their extremely premature infants may have to endure? I never felt I found the perfect approach, other than giving the statistical odds of survival and outcomes; I could not tell which babies would perform normally five, ten years later. Every parent tends to be optimistic and thinks that their premature baby will do better than expected and develop normally. I was surprised when a baby I delivered who just barely weighed over 750 grams (i.e., 1.65 pounds) developed without any physical or cognitive deficits and was even ahead of the milestones for her age. What makes some babies do so well? Is it an outcome of *nature,* that is genes, or *nurture,* with advances in medicine, the environment, or most likely a combination of both? Nonetheless, we should not underestimate the emotional stress of carrying a pregnancy with the threat of premature delivery hanging over the mother day and night.

My Niece's Story: The Impact of Prematurity on the Family

In 1982, our family experienced and understood the stress of having a premature baby. My husband's brother, Mike, and his wife were living in Rockford, Washington. My sister-in-law was pregnant with her third baby. Her two previous pregnancies had been healthy, and she had delivered at full term. During the third pregnancy, at 28 weeks' gestation, the membranes ruptured, and she immediately went into labor. She was fully dilated when she arrived at the hospital. In Rockford, the hospital was a Level 1 center with no neonatal intensive care unit to support this very premature baby. Immediately after the delivery, the baby, who weighed 2 pounds and 8 ounces, was airlifted to a hospital with a neonatal intensive care unit in Spokane, Washington. When my brother-in-law called about the early delivery and the transfer of the baby, my husband and I, knowing what the consequences could be, were worried about the short and long-term outcome of the baby, while at the same time managing not to express our concerns for the baby to my brother-in-law and his wife.

During my niece's early years of development, I was relieved to see she was developing appropriately and meeting all the milestones. I was happy to see when Rekha flourished during her school years and went to Tufts

University in Boston. Later she continued to move forward by attending Newhouse School of Communications (Syracuse University) and eventually working for CNN. It was seven years after her birth that I finally believed she was going to be okay. It was a miracle my niece had developed normal, unscathed from the physical or cognitive deficits, without the advantages of receiving steroids or a pulmonary surfactant.

I also know of babies born under similar circumstances which, unfortunately, had significant handicaps. The combination of genetics, the intrauterine environment, the presence or absence of comorbid medical conditions, the availability of a neonatal intensive care unit, and the family environment of these premature babies might all play some role in their short and long-term outcomes.

It is that long journey of the unknown that parents have to endure to see if their baby will be healthy. It is a humbling experience for me, to see parents going to great lengths to give their baby the best opportunities, even when the outcomes fall short of the expectations and sometimes involve enormous sacrifices of the entire family.

B.B's Story: Underlying Depression, Concern for the Baby, and the Impact of Hospitalization

B.B was a second-time mom who was admitted to the hospital for bed rest for premature labor with cervical dilation at around 30 weeks of gestation. She received tocolytics and antenatal steroids as recommended. As expected, she was significantly concerned about going into labor at any time, at the same time, she was tired of being on bed rest. She was a very active person, and consequently, she did not like being hospitalized when she was physically feeling well. She was also worried about her other baby at home. I discussed the importance of reducing the risks of premature delivery by whatever means. I thought I also gave her all the emotional support that she needed and addressed the issues associated with the prolonged hospitalization, especially being separated from her other child at home. She was highly educated, and so I believed she understood the rationale behind her admission and the importance of bed rest. She went into labor at around 35 weeks and delivered a healthy baby. I discharged her home within a couple of days after delivery, and she went home with the baby.

Within a few days after her discharge, B.B was unable to sleep or eat, did not care about the baby, and had started hearing voices. She was in full-blown postpartum psychosis. I immediately consulted a psychiatrist, who admitted her to a psychiatric ward. I was shocked by her appearance and her total personality change from the person I had come to know. I had taken care of her for her first pregnancy, and she had done very well after the delivery in the post-partum period other than the usual post-partum blues. It is true that post-partum depression tends to be more pronounced with subsequent pregnancies, but how could this be so very different from her previous postnatal experience?

After appropriate treatment for the psychosis, during counseling, she expressed how resentful she had been of her hospitalization and how frightened she felt about the possibility of delivering her baby early. She had thought she would be responsible if she had the baby soon for not wanting to be on bed rest. She thought she was not a good mother for not wanting to follow the instructions. It was possible she had underlying depression, but also had excellent coping skills until she experienced the stress of hospitalization during this pregnancy and fear of having a premature baby. B.B understood the importance of preventing early delivery to have a healthy baby. However, at the emotional level, she had difficulty coping with the demands and stress of pre-term labor. I was unable to recognize the impact that the hospitalization had on B.B and, consequently, failed to address her emotional plight in dealing with this pregnancy. It is not possible to know if we could have avoided her post-partum depression or psychosis, even If I had been able to address her fears better than I did and met her needs.

I am not sure if the stress triggered her full-blown psychosis or could it be a natural progression of undiagnosed depression. Postpartum psychosis is a complex diagnosis which could end up with dyer outcomes; I was glad she did well with no harm to herself and the baby. B.B taught me the complex emotions women experience during a prolonged hospitalization.

My Story: Connecting Mind, Body, and Spirit

The year 1994 was the most challenging year of my life. In June of 1994, I started experiencing sudden feelings of dizziness, the sense of a lump in my throat that I was unable to clear, and mild surges in my heart rate up to 130. I felt like I might be dying. I went to see one of my good friends, Dr. Anty Lobo, for an evaluation. My EKG was abnormal, but the stress test, including the stress echocardiogram, were normal. I went to a cardiologist for further evaluation, who placed me on Toprol, a beta blocker, to regulate my heart rate and scheduled me for cardiac catheterization. A couple of days before the planned cardiac catheterization, I felt significantly dizzy, so my husband called for an ambulance, and they took me to the emergency room at Providence Hospital. My friend and physician, Dr. Lobo, came to the emergency room around the same time I arrived at the E.R and my cardiologist, Dr. Miller, came to see me within an hour to evaluate me. For the first time, I experienced what it is like to be a patient in a hospital setting. The staff was friendly while they were performing the routines like drawing blood and hooking me up to the monitor, and yet I felt all alone, even though my husband and my physician were right there with me.

My cardiologist admitted me to the CCU in the hospital and preponed the cardiac catheterization to the next morning. There was no way I could go to sleep with wires coming off from the leads attached to my chest. I could empathize with every one of my pregnant patients who had to be on continuous monitoring with a belt placed around her pregnant belly for hours on end, sometimes for a couple of days during the induction of labor with Pitocin. It is routine care for us when we prescribe it, but nothing is customary for the patient. It is so routine that we forget to extend a word of understanding.

The next morning, I was taken to the cardiology lab to have the cardiac catheterization. As my cardiologist was giving me real-time information that all my major arteries looked very normal, I felt very dizzy, and at the same time, he noticed my heart rate dropping to 25 beats per minute, suggesting severe bradycardia. He gave me atropine to bring my heart rate back to normal. I responded to the medication immediately. I had more tests to rule out cardiac arrhythmia, which were normal. I was kept in the hospital for another two days for observation. As a patient, I felt emotionally vulnerable, not in control, and I had a hard time not having an explanation for why I had experienced severe bradycardia. I felt emotionally isolated in spite of the excellent care I received from my physicians and the staff. During my hospital stay, I wondered how it must have been for my patients when they were hospitalized, confused and concerned for their health, if I, as a physician, felt emotionally drained after my own experience. I wanted to go home, and my physician agreed with that plan. I was placed on medications to stabilize my heart rate. Even with the medication, however, I was not feeling any better.

I went to see my cardiologist one week later for a follow-up. He was excellent and listened to my concerns. Could it be that the bradycardia that I experienced was a vasovagal response to the catheterization that could be entirely different from my original symptoms? I had seen some of my patients experience a vasovagal reaction from pain with minor procedures. After discussion with my cardiologist, we decided to stop all medications and explore the possibility that I could be suffering from panic anxiety attacks. I could not believe I would be experiencing panic anxiety attacks. I was not sure why or what could be triggering them. I have always been against jumping into taking any medications. However, I knew to be functional I needed to be on anti-anxiety medication. My physician suggested it would be a good idea to be evaluated by a psychiatrist, so I went to see a psychiatrist once, who was not a big help but agreed with the diagnosis of panic anxiety attacks and gave me a prescription for a low dose of Xanax.

I continued to work with no impact on my ability to provide patient care or in my decision-making process that was noticeable to my partners or colleagues. I wanted to be off the medication and be able to control my panic anxiety attacks. During this time, I thought about all the patients who had overcome their pain during labor and were able to have a controlled vaginal birth with the Lamaze breathing technique, biofeedback and by practicing the tenets of mind, body, and spirit. I wanted to focus on practicing biofeedback by training my mind over my body with spiritual centering.

To do that, I first had to believe that nothing was physically wrong with me. Second, whenever I felt a panic anxiety attack coming on, I used biofeedback to send positive messages to my mind that nothing was wrong with me physically. I also learned to practice deep breathing techniques during the attack, the same way my patients practiced breathing during labor pain and childbirth.

Over a period of one year, I was able to control my panic anxiety attacks enough to wean off and eventually stop the medication. My patients have taught me so much, and in this situation, their examples helped me to adopt a holistic approach, rather than being on medication for my entire life. If I had not had the privilege of working with my patients in the birthing center, I am not sure if I would have learned the role of biofeedback or the connections between the mind, body, and spirit, which helped me to resolve my debilitating panic anxiety attacks.

Friends Become Family

My primary care physician and friend, Dr. Athanasius (Anty) and his wife, Dr. Kamlesh Kumari-Lobo, an OB-GYN, helped me and supported me through the most challenging time of my illness. I do not know how I would have gotten through this period without their love and support. They adopted my husband and me into their family. Anty Lobo and Kamlesh Lobo are East Africans. Kamlesh was born in Tanzania, and Anty was born in Kenya, but both are of Indian origin. They went to the same medical school, fell in love, and got married. They decided to move to the U.S. within a few months of getting married. They joined Providence Hospital in 1971 as resident physicians. Dr. Kamlesh Kumari-Lobo was three years senior to me. I knew Dr. Kamlesh Lobo as my chief resident when I was an intern and joined Dr.Connie Tubbs in private practice. Dr. Athanasius Lobo is an internist, a few years senior to me and worked as an ER physician for his first few years after graduation. In 1978, he decided to go into private practice, the same year that I joined Dr. Otlewski in private practice. Anty Lobo is an excellent, caring physician, whom I referred many of my patients, besides choosing him as my physician.

We had a few mutual friends, and Dr. Connie Tubbs was one of them. Due to such friendships, the Lobos started to include my husband and me in their get-togethers. They have two children, Ekta and Remy. In 1984, we moved into a new house in the same subdivision the Lobos had lived since 1982. We enjoyed each other's company and visited them often, becoming very close to them and their children. Anty and Kamlesh are two of the most generous people we know. We spent many holidays together and also went on a few vacations. They always shared their children's lives by letting us participate in family events without any reservations. We shared many ups and downs together. They were there for us when we needed them during my anxiety attacks and my later experience with neuropathy.

Their concern and support are something that I can never forget for the rest of my life.

Ekta and Remy became more than the children of friends; they became part of our family, and we became theirs. Ekta and Remy became very accomplished adults. Ekta is a kind, emotional, and very caring person, married to a good man, Charles Wilcox. Ekta and her husband, Chuck, made us part of their family too, and they include us for all the family events and holiday dinners. Ekta and Chuck have three beautiful daughters Natalie, Lily, and Chelsea, who give us such a pleasure and love. It is a great joy of ours to be part of their lives. Remy's kindness and his quiet, but simple caring ways, are always evident in everything he does no matter how far apart we lived. He recently married to Denise and was blessed with a baby boy a year later. We are just beginning to know his family.

We are so grateful to Kamlesh and Anty for coming into our lives, for their generosity, love, friendship, and support every step of the way. They have been there for Vinay and me through thick and thin and welcoming us as a part of theirs and children's lives. We love them from the depths of our hearts.

During the developmental years of my practice, I was fortunate also to have the friendship of one of my colleagues, surgeon Dr. Sumet Silapaswan, and his wife, Elaine. Dr. Sumet was a few years senior to me at Providence Hospital, and as a resident, I assisted Dr. Maicki during the birth of their first baby, Cherie. I came to know in later years that he had completed a one-year fellowship in head and neck cancer surgery.

He is an excellent clinician and one of the most respected surgeons at Providence Hospital. Not surprisingly, he became one of the busiest surgeons and was the primary surgeon to whom I referred most of my patients who had needed his expertise. I was thankful to have Dr. Sumet guiding my patients when faced with the devastating diagnosis of breast cancer. Besides, Sumet and his wife Elaine became our good friends. We got to know their children, too, and it has been our pleasure to watch all three of their children, Cherie and the twins Marissa and Andrew, grow up to be very accomplished adults.

My Health: A Repeat Lesson

In 1996, for a whole host of reasons, Dr. Maicki, Dr. Boutt, and I became employees of Providence Hospital. By the end of 1998, eight OB-GYN physicians were part of our group. Every one of them was an excellent physician. Practicing with a large group took away the personal relationship between the patient and the physician who was delivering them. Yes, we had less frequent night calls, but when we were on duty, we were busy running between making rounds, seeing patients on the floor, and doing many deliveries due to being part of such a large group. I was not happy and felt less joy in practicing within the confines of such a large group created.

In 1997, I began experiencing some episodes of the nonspecific symptoms of tingling with paresthesia (i.e., sharp "electric shock" sensation), resulting in numbness in the fingers of my right hand. My primary care physician and friend, Dr. Anty Lobo, referred me to Dr. Noseworthy, the chief of neurology at the Mayo Clinic, for an exam and diagnosis. Dr. Noseworthy was fabulous, spending close to 45 minutes talking to me about my symptoms, my practice, and my background. My MRI was normal. Dr. Noseworthy diagnosed me with right hemi-anhidrosis (which is the inability to produce sweat) and said that it could be contributing to my symptoms of neuropathy. He advised me that reducing the stress in my life, particularly in my practice, might help. Dr.Noseworthy also said that it was possible I might continue to feel the symptoms of tingling and numbness with mild, benign neuropathy, but with no consequence. He assured me my condition was not multiple sclerosis, which had been my primary concern.

I am so thankful to Dr. Noseworthy for taking the time to talk to me. I decided to follow through and took his advice by reducing the stress in my practice. His guidance reaffirmed my decision to move on, and I decided to stop the practice of obstetrics at the end of 1998. I decided to continue to practice gynecology, in which case I could give that one-on-one care I so desperately wanted to do, which was the most emotionally satisfying part of practicing medicine for me.

Having made the decision at the beginning of 1998, and I wanted to ensure a smooth transition. I began informing my patients, physician associates, and the hospital administration about my decision. I decided to continue to share office space with the same group but chose to take call for my patients. I felt happy about my decision and satisfied that I had closed the chapter of practicing obstetrics with the appropriate notification to all my patients. I delivered my last baby on December 17, 1998. It was an ending of one of the most important chapters in my life. I knew I would certainly miss not being part of the most emotional and joyful event in a woman's life. Like the famous saying, "When the door closes, a window opens," I was looking forward to going through that window to forge ahead in my life.

From January 1999 to 2002, I was practicing in the same office with the same group of physicians, but in late 2002, I felt I could better serve my patients in a solo practice. Along with the administration's approval, I prepared to move to a new office with a dedicated staff of my own in early 2003.

A Story of Unconditional Love

Before I moved to my new office, I had planned to visit my mother in mid-February of 2003. Since my father's death in 1989, she had visited me in the U.S. once, in 1991. From 1999, after stopping obstetrics, I had made sure I visited her frequently, about every six months to a year. She had difficulty moving on after my father's death. My sisters did all they could to support my mother, and I was grateful my sisters were there to see her through her difficulties. My mother had always been frail and had many health challenges. Since she had been in her mid-50s, I used to pray to God to keep her healthy so that I could have more time with her. In spite of her health, she remained mentally sharp, and I continued to have enjoyable and lengthy talks with her on a weekly basis. Every year that I visited her, she had become weaker, having lost her will to live after my father's death. The year before beginning my solo practice, in 2002, when I went to visit my mother, she no longer had any real quality of life, as she was mostly bedridden and was less interested in her surroundings or carrying on any extended conversations. For the first time, I accepted my mother's mortality. I remember talking to my sisters about my conflicting emotions, that I did not want her to die, while at the same time, I did not want her to live either. One of the most brilliant women I know, my mother, whom I loved so much was no longer the same; she was living but lifeless.

Just two weeks before my planned visit to India to see my mother, on February 1st, 2003, I received a call from my younger sister stating my mother had not looked well the night before. While we were discussing whether she should take her to the hospital, my mother quietly passed away in the next room in the presence of my brother-in-law, my younger niece and with one of our closest family friends holding her hand. When my mother died, my grief and the emptiness I felt was so profound; it is still hard for me to explain. What made it all worse was not having had the chance to say goodbye to my beloved mother, my guide, my teacher, and my friend.

The date of my mother's death was February 1st, 2003, and by the Indian calendar, this was the same day my father had died fourteen years earlier. It also happened to be toward the end of the month of the holiest days in the Indian calendar.

My mother always said she wanted to die during the holy days because according to *Mahabharata,* the Hindu scriptures, those who die during the sacred time would go directly into God's hands. The only thing that gave me comfort was knowing that she was in a better place and that she chose the time when she wanted to die and be with God. Accompanied by my husband, I went to India to be with my sisters and the rest of my family immediately after my mother's death so that I could participate in the ceremonial farewell to my mother.

With a heavy heart, I returned home to the U.S., for the first time feeling like an orphan. It has been fifteen years since my mother died, and there are not many days I do not think about her or miss her. I am utterly honored to be my mother's daughter, and for having had this beautiful woman in my life as my mother. That feeling has never gone away, but life has a way of pushing forward, and I found myself starting my new solo practice in April of 2003.

Gynecology and Gynecologic Surgery

"Progress is impossible without change and those who cannot change their minds cannot change anything.

--- George Bernard Shaw

Obstetricians and gynecologists belong to one of the unique specialties which deal with a whole range of concerns affecting women during the entirety of their lives. During the teenage and young adult years, the primary focus is on education to prevent sexually transmitted diseases and pregnancy. In the past three decades, the HPV virus, which is sexually transmitted, has been implicated as the causative agent for cervical cancer. Within the last two decades, a vaccine has been developed to prevent the most common types of HPV virus to decrease the risk of precancerous and cancerous conditions of the cervix. The HPV vaccination and HPV testing are a perfect example of "an ounce of prevention is worth a pound of cure."

We are the only specialty where the physician is considered both a primary-care physician and a specialist. OB-GYNs have a special relationship with their patients by providing a continuum of care from their teenage years through their senior years.

In medicine, irrespective of the specialty of practice, two of the essential components of the patient evaluation include capturing the history intake from the patient and performing a complete physical exam.

Patient History and the Physical Exam: Lost Arts?

As OB-GYNs, we have a responsibility to obtain the entire history of the patient and perform a complete physical exam to be able to care for a woman as a whole person. One of the critical aspects of practicing medicine is the art of taking a patient's entire history, which could save many lives. As an OB-GYN practicing for over 30 years, I observed the increasingly decreased focus on taking a patient's history and performing an adequate physical exam. We have become so specialty-oriented that some physicians became less focused on the intake of comprehensive patient history and instead just focused on the history of the organ system for their specialty. Our body is not disconnected the same way in which our healthcare has divided into specialties. Specialty training certainly helps us to focus on broad understanding and diagnose diseases specific to a particular organ system. It does not mean we should leave all the essential learning of human body behind. For optimal outcomes, the physician must intertwine the patient's history into the diagnosis and treatment of the health condition affecting the patient.

In 1999, I was appointed as the director of the OB-GYN Resident Academic clinic by my chairman Robert Welch. I continued in that role until 2010, when I became chief of gynecology but continued to be a teaching faculty member until I retired in 2016. Our residency program had 20 residents, admitting five residents per year. Residency programs allow significant time for training residents on managing the patients in an acute care setting in the hospital. In our hospital, each OB-GYN resident is also scheduled for four hours per week in the continuum care clinic to follow his/her patients during their four years of residency, supervised by five faculty members. This four-hour-a-week exposure in this outpatient setting gave the residents good experience following their obstetrical patients. However, it only provided a baseline understanding of clinical gynecology issues.

I was keen on educating the residents on the importance of comprehensive history intake. For example, the family history can help us to identify an at-risk population with inherited disorders like certain cancers and thrombo-embolic diseases (blood clots, heart attacks, and strokes). Knowing the family history can make a difference in how we deliver care to our patients. This critical tool, the history intake, in its entirety, is considered 80% of our diagnostic process.

I developed a three-page preprinted form for patient history. Residents felt burdened with this change but were required to follow the format. To my surprise and disappointment, one of the young faculty members, who was very involved in the resident education also resisted the change, and we had to compromise. He only changed his mind a couple of years later, after he attended the CREOG and APGO meetings where they adopted a detailed history intake, similar to what I had developed. It is a small example of how hard it is to make any changes.

The process of proper history intake and a thorough physical exam helps us to decide what tests are appropriate to aid in the diagnosis and treatment of the patient's clinical condition. In many of our department M & M (Mortality and Morbidity) conferences, I was disappointed whenever I learned that physician used technology (i.e., a test) after just listening to the patient's chief complaint and gathering only minimum history. In some cases, the physician never touched the patient or performed a complete exam. Such physicians missed the opportunity to make a crucial link to the patient's diagnosis, through a detailed history and the physical exam. Together—the history and exam— should serve as the lynchpin to help us to decide what the next step should be in the evaluation of the diagnosis and the treatment. When the evaluation process is incomplete, we might fall short of providing the patient with the most optimal care.

The most important part of taking a history is making the patient feel comfortable. In my office, I had a couch and two chairs, but no desk in between, which would have created a barrier between my patients and me. I felt it helped me to get more detailed information. Patients tend to remember better in a less threatening, comfortable setting and give better history. I got to know them better through this process, and hopefully, they got to know and trust me better.

The Cases of B.B, M.M, and U.U: Patient History-Intake and a Physical Exam Made a Difference

B.B was a 50-year-old woman, who came to see me for a routine gynecology exam, which was her first exam with me. She was one of the directors at our institution. During my history intake, I learned she had no gynecology complaints, but her medical history revealed hypertension and high cholesterol, both of which were well controlled. She was also obese. She was under the care of one of our very good cardiologists. During our conversations about her family history, she said her sister had died of a brain hemorrhage from a ruptured cerebral aneurysm at the age 32, and another family member had had the same problem. Her physician never evaluated B.B for a cerebral aneurysm. During her exam, I found a large pelvic mass, which was confirmed by an ultrasound of the pelvis. It was imminent I perform surgery to rule out a malignancy.

I advised her to get medical clearance for the surgery and suggested to her cardiologist that she may need an MRI and an MRA to rule out the possibility of a cerebral aneurysm, as I was aware certain cerebral aneurysms could be genetic. Her cardiologist was not offended by the recommendation coming from a gynecologist (which is a sign of an excellent physician), and he ordered the MRI and MRA. The MRA showed two cerebral aneurysms. The neurosurgeon felt the aneurysms were small enough just to be followed by observation.

I performed the surgery and found her tumor to be benign. However, within a year of observation, the aneurysms grew. Ultimately, her neurosurgeons treated her with an endovascular coil for one of the aneurysms, but for the other, she needed open-brain surgery. She is alive and doing well, except for mild residual cognitive changes from her open-brain surgery. It was an example of teamwork, which may have saved this patient's life. What helped this patient's outcome was for me not to ignore her family history, as well as her cardiologist not to ignore my suggestion to the patient to have an MRI and MRA. Anyone of us can miss specific points in patient history. I want to say to all the young physicians; don't leave it to the others to discover, which can lead to missing important information by everyone. Don't forget to do detailed patient history-intake.

Sometimes we get lucky. M.M was one of those cases. M.M was a 42-year-old who was transferred to me from a retiring OB-GYN for her routine gynecology exam. She had two children and was on birth control pills to prevent pregnancy. During the history intake, I learned she had had an ovarian cystectomy, and her family history revealed two of her sisters had blood clots in the legs (DVT). I tested her for the inherited genes for thrombophilia (increases the risk of blood clots). Her results came back positive for one of the enzymes, protein S antigen deficiency.

M.M was lucky; she had never developed blood clots in her legs or lungs, nor had she had a heart attack or stroke, all of which she was at higher risk for; during her pregnancies, her surgery or when taking birth control pills. Being aware of her risk factors, helped us to prevent complications when she had to undergo major surgery for endometrial cancer. She recovered well from her surgery. I am pleased to say; she is a survivor of endometrial cancer. The information from the test helped us to understand her inherited gene and to develop prevention strategies when she was in at-risk situations. The analysis also helped us give guidance to her children about following their genetic inheritance and the importance of testing. Detailed family history matters.

U.U was another patient in her 30s when she first came to see me for her routine gynecology visit. She was referred to me by my colleague, a maternal-fetal medicine specialist, after delivering her twins. After a few years of seeing her, during her physical exam, I noticed a very loud heart murmur, which I never heard before. I was no cardiologist, but I knew this murmur was abnormal. The rest of her exam was normal, and she was asymptomatic. I informed U.U of my findings regarding the heart murmur and her need to see a cardiologist. She said she was not worried, as she had a history of mitral valve prolapse and a mild heart murmur. I explained to her that the heart murmur I detected was louder than her previous murmur, and it was essential to see a cardiologist.

She went to see two pre-eminent cardiologists, one in each of two renowned hospitals. Further cardiac testing revealed that she had significant mitral-valve regurgitation with the complex valvular disease, and her cardiologists told her that she might not live beyond six months. She decided to go to the Cleveland Clinic and found a physician who was an expert in repairing the valve affected by her condition.

Surgery was successful, and she is alive and well, and it had been ten years since surgery, and her twins are now teenagers. If I had performed the gynecology exam only including breast and pelvic exams and Pap smear, I would have missed the heart murmur. I do not know if she would have survived it or not, but I was glad I listened to her heart that day. She was young and had no other primary-care physician. Gynecologists need to remember that they are primary-care physicians, too.

It is not my intent to gloat but to reiterate the importance of educating our interns and residents that the details of history intake and the physical exam matter. As healthcare providers, it is essential to remind ourselves to treat each woman as a whole person and not look at her in the narrow view of our specialty.

When Gynecology Conditions Require Surgery

Different gynecology conditions affect women in different decades of their lives, and while we can manage some medically, others require surgery. As a specialist, an equally important responsibility of the OB-GYN physician is performing operations for conditions affecting the female reproductive organs. The unique bond of an established lifetime relationship between the patient and the physician allows an OB-GYN to help a patient navigate the emotional, as well as the physical, challenges when surgery is required.

When I started my residency in 1975, we hospitalized women for 7 to 10 days after an abdominal hysterectomy. In the past two decades with the improved understanding of pre-op and intra-op care, infection prevention, early feeding, early ambulation, inspiratory spirometry, patients are discharged home within 2-3 days for the same procedure with better outcomes than in the past. Prolonged hospitalization is not always in the best interest of patients which itself can contribute to increased risk of hospital-acquired infections and other complications. Conditions that may require surgery include benign symptomatic conditions affecting the uterus and ovaries, like symptomatic uterine fibroid tumors, abnormal bleeding, endometriosis, ovarian tumors or cysts, utero-cervical vaginal prolapse, urinary stress, and stool incontinence. Certain pre-malignant conditions and all malignant conditions require surgery.

Not all gynecologists perform all operations; it depends upon an individual physician's expertise. Also, some cases may require a subspecialist's expertise. Making the decision, as a physician, to perform surgery on a patient can be very complicated. Different patients pose different challenges and requirements. The reluctance of some patients to have surgery contributes to this complexity and can be challenging, requiring a significant understanding by the physician of his/her patient. In such cases, the physician needs to start with patience to decipher what is making his/her patient reluctant to have surgery. Is the reluctance could be a response to the shock of learning her perfectly healthy-looking body may be harboring something abnormal, or a denial of the condition, or the fear of a confirmation of a suspected diagnosis, or the risks of surgery itself?

Deciding to go ahead with the surgery, for most patients, is a journey. They need to understand and accept the diagnosis, especially if the recommendation for surgery happens when they are feeling perfectly fine. It is difficult for them to believe anything other than being completely normal. This situation often leads patients to question their diagnosis. A physician's decision to perform surgery is further complicated by a woman's age, her fertility status, and the nature of the disease, as well as understanding the woman's needs. It is easier for women to understand the need for either medical or surgical intervention when they are experiencing symptoms from whatever problem that is afflicting them. It is much harder to convince an asymptomatic patient who has come in for a routine exam, when we diagnose a condition which requires surgery, such as the diagnoses of large tumors or complex cysts involving the ovary.

E.C, D.D, and O.O's Stories: The Unpredictability of Endometriosis

Pelvic endometriosis is one of the most challenging conditions to treat. Endometriosis is a condition where the lining of the uterus—the endometrium—becomes implanted in areas outside the uterus, in the pelvic region. The small foci of the endometrium could be implanted on the ovaries, in the pelvis, or even in distant places like the umbilicus or even the lungs. While the exact cause of endometriosis is unknown, it appears to be familial, often affecting multiple generations of women. Many pathways are implicated in why women have endometriosis. It is hormone-dependent and usually affects women of all age groups during their reproductive years, from menarche to menopause. The endometrium responds to the cyclical changes of hormones every month; when a woman's hormone levels drop, the endometrial lining sloughs off and bleeds, the expression of which is the menstrual period. In patients with endometriosis, the cyclical changes in hormones result in microbleeds of the endometrial implants inside the pelvis, which has no openings to drain the blood. A pigment in the blood, hemosiderin, causes an inflammatory reaction involving the surrounding tissue. Over time, this response to inflammation results in scarring of the tissue and the organs in the pelvis including the uterus, tubes, ovaries, bowel, and bladder. When ovaries are involved, in some cases it results in ovarian cysts filled with blood, commonly known as "chocolate cysts."

The difficulty with diagnosing endometriosis is its wide range of symptoms, to being completely asymptomatic. The degree of endometriosis can vary from what is known as "stage one" which involves minimal endometrial implants to "stage four" with severe adhesions from scarring which involves all the critical structures around the uterus, ovaries, fallopian tubes, bowel, bladder, and ureter, distorting the pelvic anatomy. Severe endometriosis is one of the most challenging surgeries in gynecology.

The symptoms of endometriosis may include painful periods, pelvic pain, dyspareunia (painful sex), and abnormal bleeding, or painful bowel movements. Not everyone with endometriosis is symptomatic, and not everyone with these symptoms has endometriosis. These symptoms could lead to a presumptive diagnosis, but only the surgical procedure, laparoscopy, is ultimately the path to a confirmation of the diagnosis.

Endometriosis, a disabling condition for many women, can also result in infertility. Most younger patients with the symptoms of endometriosis can be empirically treated for symptoms with various hormonal agents to suppress the ovulation. It is essential to prevent the microbleeds, which can be accomplished by stopping a patient's periods with the use of continuous birth control pills, a Depo-Provera injection, or a Merina IUD (hormone IUD). Some patients with significant symptoms are treated with medications like

Lupron that result in temporary menopause. If the symptoms continue, a laparoscopy procedure should be performed to confirm or rule out the diagnosis of endometriosis. The cauterization or excision of endometrial implants is also vital during the laparoscopy, followed by medical treatment to suppress ovulation and periods. The majority of patients with endometriosis do well with the maintenance hormone therapy and can go on with their life including having children if so they desire. Young women who continue to have pain wonder about the future of their fertility and end up dealing with a significant emotional toll.

E.C made an appointment for a routine gynecology exam and to discuss contraception as she was getting married in a couple of months from the visit. She had no complaints. During the physical exam, I felt bilateral ovarian masses, which were confirmed by ultrasound to be large complex ovarian cysts. It was one of the more complicated situations when I had to notify E.C, of her diagnosis, who was in the midst of planning her wedding, a lifetime event about which every young woman dreams. During the preoperative counseling, in the presence of her fiancé and her parents, who were present by her choice, I openly discussed the possible surgery and that our goal was just to remove the ovarian cysts and to preserve her ovaries. However, I could not guarantee the outcome of saving her ovaries, a decision I would make during the surgery. Everyone with a planned elective surgery goes through an expected anticipatory anxiety, but this patient had to go through this period with the added burden of worrying about her fertility before she was even married.

No amount of emotional support could alleviate the doubt, the fear, and the anxiety about her womanhood and the relationship with her future husband. During her surgery, I discovered she had Stage 3 endometriosis with large ovarian cysts filled with blood and with severe scarring causing adhesions. Fortunately, I was able to remove the cysts, release the adhesions, and excise most of the endometrial implants while preserving her ovaries.

E.C recovered from the surgery well and had a beautiful wedding day, just as she had dreamed and planned. I advised her to think about starting a family as soon as possible. E.C and her husband decided to attempt to get pregnant immediately. I was so happy for her when I learned that she had gotten pregnant on her honeymoon. Nine months later, she had a baby with no complications and subsequently had one more child. These are the occasions, as a physician, I felt fulfilled in making a difference. That is, one of the compelling reason why one becomes a physician, "to make a difference."

One of my patients, D.D, had been attempting to get pregnant for a few years. All the non-invasive fertility tests of the couple came back normal. As a final step in the diagnosis of infertility, I performed a laparoscopy for D.D and diagnosed her as having stage 4 endometriosis, which led to the appropriate follow-up surgery. Given her desire to get pregnant, I referred D.D to one of the top fertility specialists in Michigan for further treatment. After a few years of therapy, her fertility specialist told she might never get pregnant, and that adoption was her only choice. I remember D.D's struggle, her understandable emotional meltdowns, and our conversations during that time. It was in the early 1980s, before in vitro fertilization, and there were limited options. D.D and her husband, though disappointed, decided to move forward with the adoption and were able to adopt a baby boy.

A few years later, she made an appointment to see me because she had missed a period. Though it was unlikely she was pregnant with her previous history of severe endometriosis and infertility, a pregnancy test was performed, which is a mandatory test when a woman misses a period. Low and behold, her pregnancy test was positive! I could not believe she had become pregnant, knowing how severe her endometriosis was; and after all that fertility workup and treatment to no avail. However, now I had a new worry; she is at high risk for tubal pregnancy because of her endometriosis and the extensive scar tissue in the pelvis. I was also concerned about the risk of miscarriage, which is higher in patients with endometriosis. I hoped that this would be a healthy pregnancy, and D.D would not be robbed of the joy after she had experienced the gift of pregnancy. D.D's pregnancy was healthy, and she delivered a beautiful baby girl. It is difficult to describe the joy of parents when such a miracle happens in their lives.

O.O came to see me in her 30s with symptoms of pain with periods, dyspareunia, and pelvic pain. During her exam, I diagnosed her as having an ovarian cyst, which was confirmed by an ultrasound of the pelvis as a complex ovarian cyst. She had been trying to get pregnant for a few years, but she decided not to have any treatments to enhance her chances to get pregnant unless it happened spontaneously. During a laparotomy, I confirmed the diagnosis of stage 4 endometriosis. I had to remove one ovary during the surgery and explained to O.O that severe endometriosis, was most likely the cause of her infertility. I also informed her that some women could get pregnant, despite severe endometriosis. O.O and her husband were comfortable with adoption. They adopted a baby boy and never looked back. She never got pregnant.

The emotional ups and downs, the struggles and fears that patients go through when their fertility hangs in the balance, as they wonder if their wishes of becoming parents will ever come true were never lost on me.

After being in practice for 38 years, I am still in awe of the mystery of creation and why different patients respond differently to similar diseases/conditions. What enabled E.C to get pregnant immediately after surgery, whereas D.D had no response to a similar operation for the same disease, but then was able to get pregnant spontaneously after many years, when she was least expecting it. How does the stress of wanting to get pregnant change the physiology and create a dynamic not conducive to pregnancy? On the other hand, O.O never did get pregnant after surgery. The miracle and the genius of God's creation, beyond our understanding of science, never ceased to surprise me. Science can take us only so far, and then events happen that science cannot explain; that is why we refer to medicine more as an "art" than science.

C.Y and G.N's Stories: Diagnosis, Denial, and Acceptance

People tend to trust their bodies, expecting they will know when something starts going awry. Women find it most difficult to accept when they learn of a tumor growing inside their body, but they are entirely asymptomatic. The most common such diagnosis is an ovarian tumor or uterine fibroid tumor.

I had known C.Y for many years, and I had delivered her two children. During one of her routine visits in her 40s, my examination revealed a large ovarian tumor. I explained to her the need for an ultrasound of her pelvis, which would enable me to give her further information. Ovarian cysts can be simple, and those filled with fluid are more likely to be benign. Complex ovarian cysts, containing fluid and tissue may be benign, premalignant, or malignant tumors. Solid tumors can be benign or malignant. Blood tests for the tumor markers, like CA125 and CEA, OVA1 are not always conclusive, and a CT scan may be inconclusive also in the early stages of cancer.

C.Y did not believe me when I informed her of the ultrasound findings, which confirmed a complex ovarian cyst measuring 9 centimeters. The CT scan confirmed the diagnosis of a moderately large complex ovarian mass but showed no other abnormal findings. When I informed her of the findings of ultrasound, she thought her cyst must be only 9 *millimeters*, not 9 centimeters. She thought if it were 9 centimeters, there was no way she would not have known that it was growing inside her body. When I asked her to make an appointment to discuss surgery, she did not believe she needed surgery. I was taken aback by C.Y's response. I had thought she trusted me, and we had known each other for a long time. How could she question my recommendation, knowing what was at stake? At the same time, I understood that denial, shock, and disbelief are the first and loudest emotions displayed by many patients. I talked to her about the importance of making an appointment and, if possible, to bring her husband along. My office staff knew that all the surgical consultations get the last appointment of the day, which allowed me to spend time explaining the findings and the reasons behind my recommendation for surgery. The discussion also allowed enough time for C.Y and her husband to ask questions.

I always felt it is best to give the facts and show the patient the reports and what the tumor looked like on an ultrasound. Then I continued the conversation and provided different diagnostic possibilities, such as a benign, premalignant, or malignant tumor. It is easier to explain the findings when a patient is looking at the report, and the visual image of the report often makes the results more real to the patient. Helping the patient to accept the diagnosis is the first step in the journey toward preparing her for surgery. Patiently responding to a patient's repetitive questions helps the patient understand that you are on her side. A patient can only hear and retain about 10-20% of a physician's conversation. I learned that the repetition helps the patient to arrive at an understanding of what the physician goals are for the optimal outcomes; before, during and after the surgery.

I talked to C.Y and her husband about the hopeful findings based on the CT scan report of the complex ovarian mass with no other abnormalities. Since the tumor markers were negative, though not conclusive, it was encouraging and less likely to be an advanced stage of cancer. The next step in the journey of preparing for the surgery was to explain the levels of pre-operative, intra-operative and post-operative care, setting up the realistic expectations all along the way. I explained to C.Y, that, during the surgery, we would send the tumor for quick testing to guide me in what type of surgery I needed to perform. If there was any question of malignancy on the preliminary report, she would require more extensive surgery. I explained the possible surgical complications that, though rare, could happen, depending on the complexity of the case. Finally, I gave them a written informed consent to take home to read. I always saw my patients again, one week before the surgery, to go through the information one more time, and to answer any questions they might have thought of in the interim. This meeting helped my patients to be prepared for surgery while facing the possible life-altering diagnosis of cancer.

As we proceeded further into the discussion, I answered all her questions. Most importantly, I validated her emotional needs by recognizing her fear resulting from the uncertainty of the diagnosis. I then offered the suggestions for how she could work with the fear and the anxiety, sleepless nights, hope, and denial, which were all expected. During this challenging time, I wanted C.Y to know that I was there for her and we discussed the tools that she could use to manage her stress, which would be unavoidable until she received the final report. I learned that every patient responds differently and, however she reacts, there is no right or wrong way. My goal was to give each patient the support that she needed. Though the best surgical outcome would have been to discover that her large tumor was benign, C.Y was diagnosed to have a pre-malignant tumor, which, nonetheless, had an excellent prognosis. It has been more than twenty years since C.Y's diagnosis and, as of this writing, she has had no recurrence. During later conversations, she did acknowledge that she could not believe that she could have such a large tumor without knowing it. I learned that it was not about her lack of trust in *me*, but it had more to do with her confidence in her own body, believing nothing terrible could be growing inside her healthy body.

G.N, a professional vocalist, during her annual visit, mentioned that she had been experiencing some stomach problems for the past few weeks and had seen her primary-care physician, who had begun the investigative progress. G.N, like many of my patients, had been a patient of mine for many years and I had delivered her children about 20 years earlier. During the exam, her abdomen felt more swollen with a mass on one side. Her pelvic exam was difficult because of her strong abdominal muscles, and I could not rule out the presence of a pelvic mass. Pelvic exams can be challenging in the patients who are obese or with firm abdominal muscles.

I ordered a pelvic ultrasound, which showed a large complex ovarian cyst, measured greater than 15 centimeters, situated more in the abdomen because of G.N's pelvis was narrow. A CT scan showed the mass, with no other abnormalities, like enlarged lymph nodes, ascites (i.e., fluid in the abdomen), or omental thickening, any one of which would have been suggestive of advanced ovarian cancer. The blood tumor markers for cancer were negative. As I described in the case of C.Y, I discussed with G.N the different possible scenarios and the surgical steps and outcomes. G.N spent more time talking to me about her worries about losing her voice from the endotracheal tube with anesthesia if she decided to have the surgery. She appeared to have more concern about the loss of her voice instead of her possibility of having ovarian cancer. Such behavior may not make sense for others, but this was not an uncommon first reaction from the patients as denial often arises from the fear of the unknown. As she walked out from the appointment, she mentioned to my front desk staff that she did not believe in my diagnosis of possible malignancy. She thought that, perhaps, I was losing my diagnostic skills. I had to have several more conversations, both on the phone and in person, answering her questions before G.N was ready for surgery.

During the surgery, I noticed a small amount of mucin-looking material in the pelvis, outside the ovarian tumor and on and around her appendix. Preliminary testing of the tumor, while she was under anesthesia, showed a benign mucin-producing tumor. The appendix shares a similar lining to this particular type of tumor. I performed an appendectomy, as recommended when the ovarian cysts are mucin-producing. Once I removed the appendix, I could see that the appendix was slightly swollen. I was concerned with the small traces of mucin in the pelvis. The presence of the mucin in the pelvis could lead to the development of pseudo myxoma of the peritoneii. It is a rare form of cancer, which originates from the appendix or ovary and leads to the spread of the mucin into the abdominal cavity, ultimately adhering to the bowel and compromising its function. I irrigated the abdominal cavity with saline to remove any traces of the mucin. The ovarian pathology was benign, and the appendix showed a very small mucocele (mucin-producing cyst), post-surgery. However, I was bothered by the presence of these traces of mucin and discussed with our local gynecological oncologist, who advised no further action at the time, except for close monitoring.

It was not unusual for me to discuss cases with my friend from medical school, Dr. Ramana Surampudi, one of the best pathologists I know, who was working in Pittsburgh. During my weekly catch-up call, I talked to her about G.N's findings. She informed me that any mucocele of the appendix is considered malignant and the presence of mucin in the abdominal cavity suggests a mucocele of the appendix had breached the appendiceal wall. My friend mentioned that UPMC in Pittsburgh is the leading research institution in the country for pseudo myxoma peritoneii, and they were in the process, at the time, of recruiting patients for the treatment of intraperitoneal chemotherapy.

I already informed G.N that the diagnosis was benign, but I would be closely monitoring because of the presence of mucin material in her pelvis. Now, having this new knowledge, I needed to inform G.N about the need for further evaluation. One thinks physicians should know what treatments are available for all cases of rare conditions, but such information is not that readily available. The primary challenge was how I was to inform G.N about this new treatment option available to her and that she might have to travel to Pittsburgh to receive this treatment. Meanwhile, G.N was recovering well and moving forward with her life. How was I to break this news to G.N when I knew she was going to be devastated, to face again an unknown future, which involved further treatment? I do not see any physician who does not struggle with giving such news to the patient when it means changing the expected course of treatment.

I called G.N for a consultation in my office, where I informed her of the new information I had learned about her disease, my concern about the traces of mucin in her pelvis, and the possibility of developing pseudo myxoma peritoneii. Perhaps, not surprisingly, she did not believe her ears and expressed strong feeling to ignore my suggestion. Luckily, her friend and neighbor is also a physician. The two of them went through all the information I had provided independently, and G.N came to the same conclusion I had and decided to call UPMC. She was accepted as a patient at the UPMC, had one more surgery to remove any implants from pseudo myxoma and to receive the intraperitoneal chemotherapy treatment. The treatment was successful, and G.N was happy that she had made the right decision.

I was very relieved when G.N completed her treatment and most thankful to my friend, who provided other treatment options for G.N. I was also grateful that her physician friend who gave her the additional support that she needed to make the right decision. One cannot underestimate the importance of a second opinion providing an affirmation when a patient faces the difficult choices. Physicians need to get over the idea that it is all about them and not ignore the patient's need for confirmation. G.N was very appreciative of my persistence in getting all the information I could, once she realized how rare this condition of hers was. Her concern about losing her singing voice was one of her main reasons for not wanting to have surgery. She tells me, however, her voice is still great, and she continues to sing! Since this case, I have been able to help a few other patients who had mucocele of the appendix and made them aware of the particular treatment options when their surgeons were not aware of what was necessary for follow-up.

Changing Surgical Technology

For many years, the two most common surgical procedures in our specialty were dilatation-and-curettage (D&C) and hysterectomy (abdominal or vaginal, more abdominal cases than vaginal cases). We performed the D&C mostly for abnormal uterine bleeding. In the first decade or so of my practice, I used to do D&C as a "blind" procedure, which involved scraping the lining of the uterus with a metal curette after dilating the cervix. It was an adequate procedure to determine whether the uterine lining is benign, premalignant, or malignant. One of the significant deficiencies of the D&C was that it was not great—mostly just a hit or miss—for the diagnosis of uterine polyps or fibroid tumors of the uterine cavity. If a patient continued to have abnormal bleeding, we performed a hysterectomy.

In the 1980s, a new technology, hysteroscopy, was developed which allowed the surgeon to visualize the uterine cavity. The addition of hysteroscopy to a D&C, as opposed to a D&C alone, was akin to the difference between walking blindfolded versus walking with one's eyes wide open. With the advent of hysteroscopy, we were able to diagnose uterine polyps and fibroids. Instruments—microscissors, micro polyp forceps, and morcellators—were developed for the use of operative hysteroscopy procedures to remove the polyps and some submucosal fibroid tumors.

Many advancements were made to treat the patients with abnormal uterine bleeding with no obvious pathology. In the past, because of the contraindication of contraceptive pills after age 35 to control bleeding, many patients ended up with a hysterectomy. Later research in low-risk patients showed that the benefits of the Pill outweighed the risks and we prescribed it until the patient was into the early 50s. Besides birth control pills, there are many options to control abnormal periods, like the hormone intrauterine device (IUD), Depo-Provera, Lupron and to a lesser extent non-hormonal medications like Lysteda and NSAIDs.

A minor surgical procedure, endometrial ablation, was developed to control bleeding in patients with no response to the medical treatments. In the 1980s, Dr. Goldrath developed a laser treatment using hysteroscopy visualization to cauterize the endometrium (i.e., the lining of the uterus), which resulted in scanty or complete cessation of the periods. Now, most patients with a mild or moderate enlargement of the uterus no longer had to go through a hysterectomy to solve the problem of abnormal uterine bleeding with a benign pathology. After ablation, the patient could return to work the next day. Since the development of more refined third and fourth generation ablation systems, physicians perform the procedure in their office with local anesthesia. We have come a long way since the early days where the only treatment choice for abnormal uterine bleeding was an abdominal hysterectomy, a primary procedure with higher surgical risks and prolonged recovery of six to eight weeks. It was such a revolution in the practice of medicine and significant advancement in women's health!

If the hysteroscopy was the new technological invention of the 1980s, laparoscopy (or "keyhole surgery") had been the technological advancement of the 1960s. A laparoscope is an instrument with a camera head, which is introduced through a small incision of one to two centimeters around the belly button. Gynecology was the first specialty to use laparoscopy as a diagnostic procedure for the evaluation of chronic pelvic pain or persistent painful periods; to rule out endometriosis or pelvic inflammatory disease (PID). We performed a laparoscopy for minor procedures like tubal ligation and discharged the patients on the same day.

Hysterectomy and Minimally Invasive Surgery

In the 1980s, laparoscopy technology was advanced further with a video chip embedded into the camera head, which enabled surgeons to visualize intra-abdominal contents with the magnified images projected on a screen. Instruments were developed to perform intra-abdominal surgeries. With these technological advances, gynecologists were able to perform surgeries for tubal pregnancy, benign ovarian cystectomy or oophorectomy, myomectomy (i.e., the excision of fibroid tumors of the uterus), and operations for endometriosis without making a large abdominal incision on the patient. Some surgeons focused on getting trained to develop advanced skills by going through the additional training.

In 1989, Dr. Harry Reich was the first gynecologist to perform a laparoscopy-assisted vaginal hysterectomy in the USA. Though gynecology was the first specialty to perform the diagnostic laparoscopy procedures, many gynecologists did not develop the necessary skills or receive the training to perform advanced laparoscopy surgeries like hysterectomy. However, laparoscopy hysterectomy provided distinctive advantages over the traditional open operations, including less pain, less bleeding, early discharge and recovery, with high patient satisfaction. However, most physicians were unable to transition to performing the laparoscopy hysterectomies because of lack of the required advanced skills and the prolonged learning curve. I did learn to do laparoscopy-assisted vaginal hysterectomies and performed them in selective patients. Though I understood the need for minimally invasive surgery, 65% of my patients still had abdominal surgery. Fifteen years after the first laparoscopy-assisted vaginal hysterectomy, 60-75% of patients were still undergoing abdominal hysterectomy with more pain, more bleeding, a prolonged hospitalization, and recovery.

Robotic Surgery: Can This Innovation Be Cost-Effective?

The FDA approved the Davinci robot for prostate cancer surgery in 2000, and for gynecologic surgery in 2005. In 2006, I went to a conference at the University of Michigan where there was a display of the Davinci robot. One of the leaders in performing robotic gynecology surgery presented the early data of robotic surgery in gynecology. I had the opportunity to sit at the robot's console and went through the minimal training session to get a feel for this costly new tool that I knew could help further the direction of minimally invasive surgery in gynecology. Unlike operative laparoscopy, which requires a long learning curve, robot-assisted surgery was user-friendly with a faster learning curve. I could envision this technology helping many more physicians offer minimally invasive surgery as an option to more patients. This option would provide many benefits to the patient: a reduction of surgical pain, intra-operative bleeding, and surgical infection, which all allow for faster healing and patient recovery. I believed that this advance in technology would move the number of minimally invasive surgeries in a positive direction and benefit women's health.

In 2006, I presented to the administration at Providence Hospital the reasons why they should invest in this expensive new tool, which would promote women's health with so many benefits. I was very appreciative that the administrators listened to my argument and approved funding for the Davinci Robot, which could help to expand our minimally invasive surgery program and help many women. In April 2007, we acquired our first robot. During the early stages of using this equipment, we developed safety and credentialing criteria to ensure good surgical quality outcomes. So it was essential to make sure each hospital developed a strict credentialing process. When we do not follow strict guidelines, we fail our patients and our responsibility as physicians. To ensure the consistency in quality and safety, for the first two years, I, along with the leaders in the department and the chairman of the department, Dr. Robert Welch, developed a core faculty of seven physicians to perform a hysterectomy using the robot. During the first two years, the complication rate of the bladder, bowel, or ureteral injuries were low, compared to an abdominal hysterectomy. Our Robotic surgery team in the OR was one of the best, led by Cessalyn Harvey PA and Gary Thomas, the nurse team leader; that undoubtedly contributed to our better surgical outcomes.

After two years, we expanded the program to include more physicians, who were trained by the core faculty working as preceptors. By 2011, more than 50% of the hysterectomies performed were robot-assisted, and the patients were discharged home on the same day or first postoperative day. This program was responsible for helping hundreds of women have good surgical experience, even in more complex cases, with better outcomes and an earlier return to work. These savings at the workplace were never officially counted as a benefit of the expansion of minimally invasive surgery.

In 2005, national NIH data showed the percentage of the different routes of hysterectomy in the USA. The conclusion of the study was, the incidence of vaginal-22%; laparoscopy -14%; abdominal -64%. At our hospital in 2007, only 25% of the hysterectomies were performed using either the vaginal or laparoscopy route. It would have been a shame for us to continue going forward without offering the women better available options for surgery. Robot-assisted surgery was "three-dimensional," the movements of the instruments mimicked the surgeon's hands, and the surgeon was in total control of the handling of the devices. Robotic surgery was also ergonomically friendly with the surgeon seated at the console, and, additionally, it eliminated any impact of the surgeon's hand tremor on the surgery.

A major controversy that loomed large around robot-assisted hysterectomy was that it is much more expensive than laparoscopy-assisted hysterectomy without any proven advantages in outcomes. I agreed with that conclusion, except most of the gynecologists were unable to or did not have time to develop skills to perform these laparoscopy procedures. More OB-GYNs, because of its fast learning curve, helped many women to get the benefits of minimally invasive surgery.

I knew, with robot assistance, I could do very complex laparoscopy hysterectomy cases that I would not have been entirely comfortable performing with laparoscopy. Within a couple of years, I was performing about 90% of all my cases—including the very complex cases—with robot-assisted laparoscopy or vaginal hysterectomy.

By 2011, as a result of a shorter learning curve, 27 surgeons, half of our physicians in the department were performing robot-assisted hysterectomies. Four years into the robotic surgery program, I believed we needed to acquire another robot to meet the expanding role of robotic surgeries in other specialties besides gynecology and urology, such as general and bariatric surgeries. We needed another robot to keep up with the demand. The administration agreed with the need, but they were having difficulty in getting the funding.

The Vattikuti's Philanthropy

One of my friends, Mr. Raj Vattikuti, a very successful businessman in Detroit, and his wife, Padma, were philanthropists and had started a foundation which supported many causes. In 2000, they were one of the first donors to support robotic surgery for prostate cancer and had launched the Vattikuti Urology Institute at Henry Ford Hospital in Detroit. Later, they also founded the Global Vattikuti Robotic Institute to expand the applications of robotic surgery around the world.

I had known Raj and Padma since the 1970s and had helped deliver their two children at Providence Hospital. I helped bring Raj and Padma Vattikuti and Providence Hospital together to develop a joint robotic institute. Their foundation helped us with a significant donation toward the purchase of a second robot and, as a result, the Providence-Vattikuti Women's Robotic Institute was born. The partnership with the Global Vattikuti Robotic Institute opened our hospital and me to new opportunities. I had hosted the physicians from India to exchange ideas and robot-assisted surgical techniques. I was invited to speak at the Global Vattikuti Conferences. I was invited to the national annual Endo-Gynecology Conference in Calcutta, India, to perform live Robot-assisted telesurgery hysterectomy with more than 400 members in attendance. Having the opportunity to share my ideas with the professionals in India and learn about the cost-effective processes implemented in their institute was one of the highlights of my professional life. I am grateful to Raj and Padma for allowing me to be a part of the faculty of Global Vattikuti Robotic Institute.

Robot-assisted hysterectomy at Providence Hospital made a significant contribution to our program of minimally invasive surgery. However, I did understand that robot-assisted hysterectomy is more expensive than laparoscopy hysterectomy. In 2012, I started an educational project for our department using a data tool to help to reduce the costs, that looked at the instrument utilization, OR time, quality outcomes and provide the physicians with timely (blind) data measured by benchmarks.

Our goal was to reduce the cost of robotic surgery without having any negative impact on the quality. I provided every physician the cost list of each instrument utilized in our surgical procedures and discussed how to optimize the utilization of the surgical instruments during our monthly department meetings. Within two years, we had reduced the costs so much that our cost of robotic surgery was about $2000 less than the national average and within $200 of the average laparoscopy costs reported in the national data. The year after, we reduced the cost of doing robotic hysterectomy even farther. During the same period, our surgical complications decreased, most likely, a result of our surgeons gaining more experience in performing this surgical procedure. The informational project was a perfect example of; when given the right tools, information, and education, and without pointing fingers at any individual, most physicians could set their egos aside and do the right thing in reducing the costs while performing at the highest level.

If this program could be adopted nationally, such a demonstrable cost reduction would help void the cost argument while sharpening the focus on expanding the best service to the most patients. The evidence is clear that minimally invasive surgery like vaginal, robot-assisted, or laparoscopy-assisted hysterectomy should be the first options as they have lower complications and readmission rates. Despite this evidence, some surgeons still perform only abdominal hysterectomy without offering these options or an appropriate referral to their patients to someone who will.

As I look at my experience with the minimally invasive surgery with the robot-assisted hysterectomy, I felt more comfortable in operating on the patients with the more complex diagnosis. I would not have offered a laparoscopy surgery in such complicated cases just a few years ago. I am not stating that some advanced laparoscopists would not perform them, but most gynecologists that I knew were not doing them.

V.V's Story: Role of Robotics in Complex Surgery

V.V was referred to me for a surgical consult to address a significant uterine fibroid tumor of 18 to 20 weeks size, with very heavy bleeding and anemia from blood loss. She had a history of previous multiple myomectomy (excision of numerous fibroids), with open surgery. After the appropriate workup, I discussed all the different options with her. She had not responded to hormone therapy. She was not a candidate for a hormone IUD or endometrial ablation because of her enlarged uterine cavity. I discussed with her the only other non-surgical option, a uterine fibroid embolization performed in the radiology department, which is 80%-90% effective. However, the patient wanted a hysterectomy, a 100% definitive therapy. I informed V.V that her risks of surgery had increased because of the previous multiple myomectomy by an open procedure, which could have resulted in severe adhesions. Also, the possible risks with any hysterectomy, like an injury to the bowel, ureter, and bladder, could be higher because of her previous surgery. I advised her to begin iron therapy by iron infusion to improve her anemia and to reduce the risk of blood transfusion. I let her know that her moderate obesity could also increase her risk during and after the surgery.

Ultimately, I advised robot-assisted hysterectomy, which would allow me to remove her large uterus by a relatively new and safer process of internally placing the uterus in a bag and cutting it into small pieces with a knife. I explained to her that this method would ensure a reduction in the risk of spreading any occult malignancy, even though that risk was low. V.V understood the benefits and the risks. At the end of the discussion, she decided to have a robot-assisted hysterectomy. During the consultation, I addressed her anticipatory anxiety and provided her with the coping tools and pre-op instructions. However, V.V did not show up for her appointment one week before surgery to address any questions, concerns, or fears that most patients experience before surgery. I tried to call her without success. It is rare for a patient to cancel the operation, without informing the surgeon of such decision.

To decide to have surgery is hard enough even when there is a longstanding established relationship between the physician and the patient. It was hard to get into the patient's state of mind, but the thought crossed my mind if she was hesitant to place the trust in a physician, whom she hardly knew and to put faith in that physician doing the surgery. Who could blame her if she had thought that?. I sent a letter to V.V informing her of the importance of deciding on the treatment of her symptoms of bleeding and anemia, symptoms that would only become progressively worse. V.V called back about a month later and made another appointment, at which time she informed me she was frightened but was now ready for surgery. As anxiety can influence surgical outcomes, I talked with each of my patients about the importance of mechanisms to stay calm and encouraged them to find activities that create positive biofeedback.

I performed V.V's surgery, and as expected, the procedure was very involved with severe adhesive disease involving the ureter. Nonetheless, I was able to complete the operation as planned, with no complications and with minimal bleeding. V.V was discharged the very next morning and was able to get back to work just two weeks after the surgery.

She was one of the examples of several cases I performed under similar circumstances. It is impossible to know what would have been the outcome if any of these women needed to have open surgery. I would expect V.V would have been at risk; to have more bleeding, to need a blood transfusion, to a higher risk of infection, to experience more pain, to have a prolonged hospital stay, and a longer recovery. We cannot underestimate the patient satisfaction that goes along with these clinical and physical benefits, not to mention the economic benefits to society from quicker recovery and early return to the workforce.

Similar changes were happening in vaginal surgical techniques, such as those involving uterine or vaginal prolapse, and surgeries with more anatomical repair of defects rather than just the repair of the visual prolapse. I was one of the few physicians who learned the new techniques in performing pelvic organ prolapse. New minimally invasive procedures were also developed to surgically treat urinary incontinence during the time I was in practice as well.

Science and technology in medicine are continually evolving. As physicians, our willingness to learn and adapt to the changes that affect our clinical practice does make a significant difference to the patient sitting before us. These patients trust us and expect us to give them the best treatment options, which will help them to have the best outcomes. I was truly honored to be part of a department, where most of the physicians were very engaged with and adapted well to the changes in new science and technology, changes that were genuinely beneficial to our patients.

The treatment for many diseases, the surgical techniques, and the pre-and post-operative management of patients has changed so significantly during my lifetime. Thirty-eight years ago, I indeed could not have had answered correctly, if someone had asked me to prognosticate and predict the progress, in gynecologic surgery, over the next thirty-eight years. I feel privileged to be part of the significant changes in our specialty during my career. Even though I lived through this period and adapted to these changes, I am still in awe of how far we have come.

Cancer and Women's Health

When someone has cancer, the whole family and everyone who loves them does, too.
--- Terri Clark

Cancer in women is one of the leading causes of morbidity and mortality. The word "Cancer" is the most frightening word in the dictionary of human life, that every person dreads to hear when receiving a diagnosis and a challenge everyone hopes never to have to face. Cancer, due to its very nature, turns one's life upside down, halting all the hopes and plans for the future. Cancer cure rates are based on the first five years data, and not knowing what lays ahead beyond the five years lead to peoples' uncertainty. In the recent years, more data is looking at 5 to 10-year survival and the recurrence rates for certain cancers. New treatments are helping to manage cancer as a chronic disease when the cure is not possible. Majority of the people diagnosed with cancer, experience the stages of grief; denial, anger, bargaining, depression, and acceptance. It is not unusual for cancer patients to require counseling to develop coping tools to help them through the stages of grief, and treatment to combat depression. For most women living with cancer is a journey of fear to acceptance. In time, women learn to conquer the fear of death and move on to embrace the joys of life. Women with recurrent cancer, despite the level of uncertainty in life, I had seen them live courageously with an attitude to love and cherish all the little victories experienced daily.

Families of a loved one diagnosed with cancer tend to have such a varied response to the fear of losing the person that they love, which could change their lives forever. Some respond with denial, some with emotional remoteness while trying to deal with their fear and grief, and some are lost, not knowing what the right response is. It happens more often when it is the wife who receives the cancer diagnosis, and the husband ends up being the caregiver. This lifestyle is a reversal of their typical roles in the family, where in general, the woman plays the dominant role in meeting the day-to-day needs and wants of her husband and children. Most husbands are lost, frightened, and overwhelmed with their grief. It is hard for most of the spouses to emotionally manage their caregiver responsibilities while also meeting the physical demands required to support the treatment of cancer. Some husbands find it more challenging to connect with their wives, not knowing how to provide the emotional support a woman so desperately wants and needs.

Majority of the cancers are asymptomatic until later stages, which increases the mortality rates. In the last 50-plus years, we have come a long way in developing strategies for, screening, prevention and early diagnosis of some cancers. In recent years, some cancer outcomes have improved significantly, with declining death rates. However, overall mortality rates for cancer is still one of the highest, and the early diagnosis and treatment of most malignancies are challenging. Gynecologists, as primary care physicians for women play a significant role in the prevention, diagnosis, and treatment of cancers. The most common causes of malignancies in women involve the breast, lung, and colon. Fortunately, two out of these three common cancers, breast and colon, now routinely are screened with mammograms and colonoscopies, respectively. These screening procedures have improved the early diagnosis of breast and colon cancers. Any cancer, if diagnosed early, is less likely to result in death and does not need the life-threatening treatments of chemotherapy and radiation therapy. Unfortunately, very few other cancers have tests for mass screening.

V.W's Story: A Life I Could Have Saved

Cervical cancer used to be one of the leading causes of cancer deaths in women. It is a perfect example of what the simple test like Pap smear, along with more recent HPV screening, has accomplished in bringing down the death rates of cervical cancer. In the U.S., there has been a 70% drop in the mortality rate for cervical cancer, since the adoption of the Pap smear in the 1950s as a mass screening test. In developing countries, cervical cancer is still one of the leading causes of death, due to lack of mass screening. In spite of the availability of this simple screening test in the U.S.A, about 12,000 new cervical cancers are diagnosed every year, and approximately 4,000 women die annually. In the 1980s, researchers discovered that the HPV virus, a sexually transmitted disease caused cervical cancer. In 2006, HPV vaccines were developed, to reduce the risk of cervical cancer further, to be given to the girls and more recently to boys, starting at the pre-pubertal age of 9 to the adults up to the age of 26, preferably before the young women or men engage in sexual activity.

In my practice, I had very few patients who had cervical cancer, especially in those patients who received regular Pap smears per guidelines. I diagnosed many patients with the pre-cancerous condition, cervical dysplasia. Cervical dysplasia progresses slowly, usually progressing from mild to severe as CIN 1 (cervical intraepithelial neoplasia), CIN 2, and CIN 3. It takes another eight to twelve years for CIN 3 to develop into invasive cervical cancer. So, there is a long latent phase, which provides ample time to treat CIN 3 with minor surgery by excising a portion of the cervix, a procedure called cone biopsy. After having a cone biopsy, most patients with CIN 3 rarely ever develop cancer of the cervix, especially if appropriately monitored according to the guidelines.

The one person, whose life I could have saved and regret I did not, left an indelible impression on my mind that I will never forget. V.W came to see me only one time for a routine gynecology exam, which included a Pap smear. She was in early 40s at the time and had not seen a gynecologist for many years. I think she felt comfortable enough to see me because I had taken care of her pregnant teenage daughter, whom I delivered a few months earlier. V.W's Pap smear came back abnormal. She returned for her follow-up appointment to have a procedure called colposcopy, which is a microscopic examination of the cervix with a colposcope. Her colposcopy showed significant abnormal lesions, and I biopsied all the abnormal looking lesions. The biopsies revealed CIN 3, which was also present in the cervical canal. I called to inform her that she needed a further procedure, a cone biopsy of the cervix, to confirm the diagnosis and for a possible cure. I advised V.W to make an appointment to discuss these findings further. However, she did not make any further appointments. As a follow-up, I made few more calls, explaining that if CIN 3 goes untreated, she could develop cervical cancer, which could be life-threatening. I received no response from V.W I thought she was probably scared and was frightened to know any further information about the diagnosis or treatment. The denial is the most common natural human response. In desperation; I sent a letter explaining the benefits and the risks of having, or not having the procedure. I could not change her mind, and she never came to see me, in spite of my multiple efforts.

A few years later, suddenly, I got a call from her husband, wanting to talk to me about his wife, whom I had seen a few years ago. It was long before HIPPA rules when there was more leeway concerning talking to the family members. I knew who his wife was (his daughter was still my patient) and wanted to know why he wanted to talk to me. During our conversation, he explained to me that his wife's stomach was very swollen and wondered if it could be anything to do with the concerns I had had for her and the treatment she did not receive. He said she felt uncomfortable coming to see me, because of our history of her not having followed my instructions. I advised him of the need for her to see a physician because I could not weigh in on her condition, not having seen her. She was 45 years old.

I later learned from her daughter, who had seen me for her annual exams, that her mother was diagnosed to be pregnant, was well into her third trimester, but unfortunately was also diagnosed with cervical cancer. I was told she had a baby girl at around 34 weeks of pregnancy by cesarean section along with modified radical hysterectomy to treat her cervical cancer. I was not sure what was the stage of cancer, but I thought it had to be stage 2 or less for her to have surgical treatment. However, within two years after the delivery and the surgery, her cancer metastasized. V.W was never too far from my mind, a reminder of my inability to change her mind, that one life I could have saved, and I was not able to. She came to visit me along with her daughter to thank me for all that I had done in trying to help her, but there were more words left unsaid. I could only comfort her with a hug. Her courage and decision to come to see me were genuinely touching, as I was a reminder to her of how the decision not to follow my advice, founded by fear, was about to take her life. I could not imagine the burden of pain and guilt she must have felt, and how her reluctance to be appropriately treated had changed her life forever, and led to earlier death, leaving her children motherless, especially the 2-year-old.

She died within a few months after her visit to see me. Her daughter K.W. settled into adult life, got married, had one more child, and continued to see me until my retirement. Her younger sister, who became motherless at age 2, grew up with the love and support of the family and did well. V.W would be happy to know her children have made her proud by the way they lived and would allow her soul to rest in peace.

Breast Cancer: New Understandings

Breast cancer is the leading cause of death in all women between the ages 35 to 49 and is the most common cancer in women of all ages. One in eight women, 12%, develop breast cancer every year, accounting for about 250,000 new invasive breast cancers and 60,000-plus cases of pre-invasive cancer. Approximately 40,000 women die from the breast cancer annually. Gynecologists are at the forefront of screening and diagnosing breast cancer.

The success of any cancer treatment depends on the stage of cancer at the time of the diagnosis, the cancer cell type, and tumor genetics; We made significant improvements in the last 30 years concerning the early diagnosis of breast cancer. In the 1970s, we did mammograms in a limited number of cases. In the 1980s, the mammogram was recommended for regular screening with a baseline starting at age 35, routine screening at age 40, and continued screenings every 1-2 years. In the last decade, routine testing has changed to begin at age 40 and continue every 1-2 years.

Unfortunately, there is nothing simple about understanding the risks and benefits of any procedure. It is no different with the mammogram, around which several controversies swirl. One question is whether the mammograms over-diagnose early breast cancer that never would become life-threatening; or over-diagnose benign conditions which result in the need for more tests, creating undue anxiety; or whether the mammograms reduce the death rates from breast cancer. In addition to these questions, it is essential to understand that mammograms fail to detect breast cancer in about 10% to 15% of patients. Then there is the controversy over whether mammogram screening should start at age 40 or 50 and whether it should be performed every one or two years.

I performed annual screenings on all my patients starting at age 40 as per cancer society recommendations. After successfully diagnosing early breast cancers from routine screening in many women, I felt that while some cancers in the very early stage may not advance to cause death, I had no way to distinguish which patients would do well and which patients would be facing death. Hopefully, in the very near future, this challenge of determining tumor genetics and prognosis will be resolved by a liquid biopsy test, a mere blood test. As a physician at the front lines of diagnosing breast cancer with no medical consensus, I continued annual mammograms starting at age 40. Like most physicians, I was influenced by what I had seen in my practice and felt it was worth saving the life of every patient

I could. I decided not to change my practice until the controversy regarding guidelines is resolved.

Another question is when to stop doing mammograms in elderly patients. In patients expected to live less than ten years, we do not recommend routine screening because they are unlikely to die from breast cancer. What about a healthy woman in her late 70s to early 80s? It is very difficult to estimate the longevity of individuals, and recommendations are vague. My practice was not to recommend a mammogram for healthy women at age 80 unless a patient insisted on having one. I wish there were guidelines when to stop doing mammograms.

The risk assessment tools (Gail model and others) for breast cancer were developed to decipher individual risks with no history of breast cancer. We calculated the risk score with different data points that include the age of the woman, the race, the age of menarche, the age of first live birth, family history of breast cancer in 1st-degree relative, history of breast biopsies, and positive atypical hyperplasia. Separate testing guidelines were developed to identify at-risk individuals for inherited genes. The highest risk for breast cancer is when a woman carries the BRCA gene. When a family member has breast or ovarian cancer or positive BRCA gene, women and men in the family should follow the NCCN guidelines for getting tested for the gene. Women with Ashkenazi Jewish ancestry are at even higher risk for BRCA gene mutation.

BRCA gene mutation not only increases the risk of breast cancer, but it also increases the risk of ovarian cancer, which is one of the deadliest diseases in women. Other risk factors implicated in breast cancer include obesity, alcohol intake, even in moderation, and hormone therapy. The mortality rates of breast cancer have been reduced by an average of 20% over the last 20 years, with a five-year survival rate close to 90%. Most breast cancers occur randomly, but the risk increases with a family history of breast cancer, especially in first-degree relatives, even without the inherited gene

Controversy continues as to what is the cause of the reduction of the mortality rate in breast cancer. Is this decrease a result of an increase in the number of patients receiving an earlier diagnosis, or because of better treatment? There has been an increase in the incidence of breast cancer—from 8% incidence in the 1980s to 12% now—with more women diagnosed early. It is most likely the result of both *routine* screening and the advanced screening technologies of a mammogram with adjunctive 3D images, breast ultrasound, and MRI.

In the last 20 years, the mortality rate reduction in advanced cancers, a very moderate 8%, could be due to the understanding of tumor genetics and the hormone receptor status of tumors. It could be attributed to the improvements in chemotherapy, and the chemo-prevention medications, to decrease the recurrence of cancer. However, the overall decrease in the mortality rate of about 20% is most likely influenced by the higher pool of early breast cancers, some of which may never have progressed to advanced stages.

In spite of all the advances, we have more questions than answers, and our challenge is to figure out which patients are at risk of having cancers that will end up progressing to advanced stages. As we are learning—and unlearning—the science of medicine, we can only continue to treat our patients with the information at hand, which is somewhat influenced by our personal experiences as physicians. The women who went through breast cancer and died fighting it, made me think of what-ifs for the rest of my professional life.

N.N's Story: A Decade Too Early

In 1980, N.N came to see me in her late 20s because she was having difficulty getting pregnant. I gave her some guidance on how to optimize the odds of getting pregnant, and I still remember how excited she and her husband were when she became pregnant and had a healthy baby girl. A couple of years later, she was able to get pregnant again and had another baby girl. At age 32, just a few years after her last baby was born, N.N came for her routine yearly exam. During the breast exam, I felt a small lump, one centimeter in size, in one of her breasts. I reassured her that the lump was most likely benign. However, I wanted her to see a general surgeon for further evaluation, and to assess the need for a biopsy or an excision of the tumor. It was decades before the availability of ultrasound-guided or stereotactic biopsies. Interestingly, gynecologists are specialists in women's health and perform surgery, but breast surgery is a part of the general surgery specialty for reasons unknown to me and, indeed, unexplainable.

During the discussion with N.N and in response to my recommendation to see a surgeon, she stated her husband was being transferred and would be moving to the western part of Michigan, and she would see a surgeon as soon as she moved. N.N did see a surgeon within a couple of months. Considering her age and the size of the tumor, he felt it was most likely benign. However, he advised the excision of the tumor for confirmation. Unfortunately, the result came back as invasive breast cancer. He performed a radical mastectomy and full lymph node dissection, which was the standard surgical treatment at the time. Her lymph nodes were negative for cancer, and the tests for metastatic disease were negative. She returned to the area after a couple of years, when her husband was transferred back to Detroit. She was monitored closely by an oncologist. At age 36, her cancer came back with a vengeance, metastasizing to every part of her body: lungs, spine, and, eventually, to the brain. No chemotherapy helped her, but she fought with valor. She just wanted to see her two young children grow up, but lost her fight and died within two years, at age 38.

N.N's death came before our knowledge of tumor genetics, hormone receptor assay, chemoprevention, and oncogene typing to decipher the need for chemotherapy and radiation therapy. It was also before we understood that a mastectomy, in most cases, may not be any better than a lumpectomy and radiation therapy, and in selective cases chemotherapy. If N.N had been born a decade are so later, would she have survived? No one has an answer for that, but

I know she would have had a better chance of living or living longer. She is never too far from my thoughts, and I heard from N.N's best friend G.H., her children are doing well. When I think of her, I wonder what could have been if we only understood her disease better. We could not speed up the arc of progress, but my mind never stops wondering about all the what-ifs. In the end, I had to come to terms with the limitations of my ability to save lives.

F.F's Story: Living Life While Accepting Death

F.F had been my patient for many years. She was a single working woman, never married, who lived with her parents. At age 40, on her routine mammogram, there was a lesion in her breast, and a malignant tumor could not be ruled out. As we were discussing the plan of further diagnostic procedures, she mentioned that she was caring for her mother who was dying of colon cancer. Her mother also had a history of breast cancer. F.F's diagnostic biopsy showed invasive cancer. Any carcinoma in younger patients has a higher risk of recurrence. I was taken aback by how pragmatic she was in dealing with her cancer while caring for her mother who was dying of cancer. F.F went through the appropriate surgery and treatment for her breast cancer. Her mother died after F.F's treatment.

Four years later, F.F developed the local metastatic disease in one of her hips, for which she had surgery and chemotherapy. Nonetheless, she continued to work and lived with her father.

Cancer became a chronic disease for her, and over many years, she developed lesions in her lung for which she would undergo periodic chemotherapy as a palliative treatment since hers was no longer curable. She never stopped working. I advised her to have BRCA gene-testing when it became available, not for her benefit, but in the interest of her family members. When she decided against having the test, I was surprised that F.F, who was very close to her family and a caregiver, had decided against the test which may have helped other family members. It is a perfect example of the enigma of human behavior, which does not fit into a little box with a bow tied neatly around it. Four years later, F.F developed brain lesions. She never went to counseling or needed any anti-anxiety or anti-depressant medications during her entire journey with cancer, from the time of diagnosis to the end.

One evening, she called and said in her usual pragmatic way, that it was time for her to be in a home hospice care, and Angela hospice had gotten her a bed, final step in her journey facing this deadly disease. It was the first time I had ever received a call from a patient to say a personal goodbye as she was lay dying. I was lost for words like most people would be, so I said the only thing I could say; that I would pray for her to find peace and comfort during this final journey of her life.

As a physician, I was privileged to be part of F.F's valiant fight, though I was not directly involved in treating her cancer. I was profoundly touched by her thoughtfulness to call me personally to say goodbye as one would do to one's family members. Again, like many times in my life, as a physician, I felt blessed to have known many phenomenal women, who taught me and let me be a witness to a part of their journey. They showed me how to live and love, even when lingering between life and death. F.F lived every day to the fullest and decided how to live and how to die, dealing with her challenges one step at a time, without questioning. I am not sure if she ever wondered; Why me?

Many years later, I diagnosed F.F's niece with invasive breast cancer at age 26. Her gene testing for the BRCA genes was negative. The story of genes is still evolving, and while breast cancer had been linked to few other genetic diseases, still more genes are likely to be connected to inherited breast cancer. The more we think we know, there is more we have yet to understand!

H.H's Story: The Role of Genes and the Difference a Decade Made

I had seen H.H for many years and had delivered her two children. When she was in her early 40s, she came in for an appointment because she had felt a small lump in her breast. Finding a lump in one's breast is one of the most common reasons for a call to our office and is usually associated with anxiety or a fear of cancer. Our office staff knew to get the patient in, on the same day or the next day. Most tumors are benign and are merely cysts. I routinely aspirated those lumps in the office. If an aspiration yielded fluid and the lump resolved, I could immediately reassure the patient that it was benign. During the aspiration, if the lump felt firm to the needle, and if there was no fluid, I would immediately start the process of testing with a mammogram and an ultrasound of the breast. If the results showed that the lump appeared suspicious for malignancy, I would immediately refer the patient to radiology for a breast biopsy. During my many years of practice, I had seen many palpable lumps diagnosed with cancers even when the diagnostic tests of mammogram and ultrasound were negative. Patients, as well as some physicians, felt a false sense of security if the tests were negative, thinking that the lump had to be benign. I needed to remind patients that a mammogram has a 10% false negative rate. I referred all my patients with a solid, palpable lump, even with a negative mammogram or ultrasound result, to a surgeon for further evaluation. The physical exam, mammogram screening, and advanced adjunct testing all play a role in the diagnosis of breast cancer.

I examined H.H, and I felt the lump to be about one centimeter in size. I attempted to aspirate the lump but got no fluid. The mammogram and ultrasound confirmed a solid tumor, about one-and-a-half-centimeter in size. A radiology-guided biopsy was positive for invasive cancer. I let H.H know the diagnosis. Her two children were, at the time, young teenagers. Every time I had to inform any patient with the diagnosis of cancer, I was very conscious of how it was about to change her life forever and even worse for a mother of two teenagers. I tried to talk about the facts and at the same time give her hope that many women with breast cancer outlive their cancers and die from some other cause. Time is the only thing that helps a person to have less fear of death and to move forward in life. H.H's cancer was discovered to be much larger, almost five centimeters. Such a discrepancy between the exam and diagnostic testing to the surgical findings is very rare. The type of breast cancer tumor that H.H had was a lobular carcinoma, which occurs in 10% of the population. This type of tumor is difficult to palpate or to even see in the diagnostic images. Based on the surgical findings, stage of her cancer was 2B, which had changed her prognosis.

Because of the H.H's tumor size, the surgeon recommended a mastectomy followed by chemotherapy. H.H decided to go to the Karmanos Cancer Center for chemotherapy. H.H, by her nature, was not overtly emotionally expressive, which did not mean she did not go through the emotions of grief, anxiety, and fear, but she did focus on getting better. She had a strong family history of breast cancer in more than two second-degree relatives at less than 50 years of age, and her parents had no history of related cancer. After she completed her treatment and when she came to see me for her annual gynecology exam, I gave her a published article in a 2001 issue of the New England Journal of Medicine about the guidelines regarding which patients require BRCA gene testing. I gave H.H the reasons why she should be tested, discussing the high risk of breast and ovarian cancer in patients who test positive for the BRCA gene. If she were to be positive, her risk for ovarian cancer would be high, between 20 and 40%, whereas in the general population, the risk for ovarian cancer is 1-2%. If she tested positive, she would have to decide to have a mastectomy of her other breast and bilateral salpingo-oophorectomy (i.e., the removal of her fallopian tubes and ovaries) to help significantly reduce the future risk of breast and ovarian cancer. Not everyone who is positive for the gene develops breast or ovarian cancer. What makes these abnormal genes develop into carcinoma are related to gene penetrance or triggers from the environment stimulating the already defective gene. For H.H to be positive, one of her parents would have to be positive for the gene. Both men and women carry the gene, and it is an autosomal dominant gene. Men can also develop breast cancer.

H.H was not ready to have this genetic testing. The mere possibility of inheriting an abnormal gene creates such conflict in most of the women; the initial response was not to acknowledge any possibility of having an abnormal gene. The patient also begins to worry; if she were to be positive, she would be responsible for her children possibly having an abnormal gene. Though no fault of her own, most women feel guilty to be a carrier of the inherited gene. I tried to help H.H see the other side of the equation: it could be empowering to know her gene status.

I counseled many women who were at risk for the inherited BRCA gene. I explained that if she were positive for the BRCA gene, I would recommend frequent screening starting at an early age. I recommended bilateral mastectomy and bilateral salpingo-oophorectomy, which could reduce the risk of mortality from cancer of breasts, fallopian tubes, and ovaries. I discussed further that the Optimal time for surgery would be after completing woman's family needs, or any time if the patient is ready. Despite my counseling, I did not encounter too many patients who accepted my recommendation, the first-time I brought up the topic. It often took a journey toward acceptance over several years. Some patients were concerned about their health insurance, others about their life insurance, especially if the patients who were at high risk for inheriting the gene but did not have cancer. Patients who already had cancer tended to move forward with their lives but had no appetite to know any further abnormal results. It is a typical human response on display. Most patients want to forget about their cancer and have the need to move on living their life without a constant reminder of what could go wrong.

H.H is a nurse, and while she understood my explanation about why she should have the test, she was not ready. At every subsequent visit, I suggested to H.H that she consider genetic counseling and then decide whether to have the test. A couple of years after my initial recommendation, she decided to have the genetic counseling and made an appointment at the same cancer center where she had received chemotherapy. At the time, her genetic counselor felt she was a borderline candidate for genetic testing, and it was up to her to have the test or not. She did decide to have the test and was positive for the BRCA 1 gene. Unlike some women, however, she did not hesitate to have the necessary surgeries, having a mastectomy of the other breast to reduce the risk of breast cancer as well as a bilateral salpingo-oophorectomy to decrease the risk of the deadlier ovarian cancer. A few years later, her sister was diagnosed with breast cancer.

I am pleased to say she is doing well over 14 years after her initial diagnosis. She is alive to see her children grow up and fulfilled one of the dreams that every mother has, that is to see her daughter get married. Her daughter, L.H has to go through her journey, deciding whether or when to begin screening or have genetic testing. I recommended genetic testing after completing the childbearing plans unless the patient wanted to undergo early testing. I had seen L.H as my patient, and at age 25, I advised her to have initial screening with a mammogram, a semiannual pelvic exam, CA125 blood test, and a yearly pelvic ultrasound. She chose not to have any testing. L.H felt healthy, as it would be for most people, it was very hard for her to believe that she could be carrying the abnormal gene that her mother has. I hope she does not wait too long to start the screening tests.

In spite of my extensive counseling about the need for testing and the emotions involved in making these decisions, some patients declined the testing. Though I understood the fear and denial, I still struggled when a patient decided to ignore the opportunities that might be helpful in saving her life. Denial, as well as hope and optimism, is one of the most fundamental human defenses as a response to any challenge in life, I would think it is true from the beginning of times.

Ovarian Cancer: The Deadly Disease

Cancer that women think and worry about most often is ovarian cancer. Ovarian cancer is not the most common cancer, but it is one of the gynecologic cancers with the highest mortality rate. Every year, about 22,000 women are newly diagnosed with ovarian cancer, and about 14,000 women die from it. Like most other cancers, it has an excellent prognosis when diagnosed in the early stages. The challenge with ovarian cancer is its stealth nature of progression, with no symptoms, or only vague symptoms, until cancer has already metastasized to the other organs. Effective screening for early detection of ovarian cancer continues to be a medical challenge. Most of the blood tests like CA125, CEA, OVA1 or ultrasound images are limited in their scope as screening or diagnostic tests, with high false positive or false negative results. There is no clear-cut mass screening tool for ovarian cancer, unlike for some malignancies: Pap smear for cervical cancer, mammogram for breast cancer, and colonoscopy for colon cancer, all of which save many lives.

The identification of higher-risk patients was brought to the forefront when Gilda Radner, a celebrity from *Saturday Night Live,* died from the complications of ovarian cancer. She wrote a book describing her ten-month plight before she was diagnosed with ovarian cancer, which, by then, was already in an advanced stage. Gilda had a history of multiple family members who had died from ovarian cancer, and she was of Ashkenazi Jewish descent. It is difficult to know if she would have survived the disease even if her physicians diagnosed ovarian cancer ten months earlier, but her story helped to advance the discussion regarding the importance of starting a family registry to identify higher-risk patients.

Research scientists had been studying the significance of family history in ovarian and breast cancer since the late 1970s, but it still was only in the research phase. Rosewell Park Cancer Institute established the family ovarian cancer registry in 1981. It took a few more years before physicians at practice level became aware of the significance of family history. Gilda Radner's husband, Gene Wilder, was a co-founder of Gilda's Club, which became both a great resource for information and a support system for ovarian cancer patients. In the early '90s, it was well-known fact that Gene Wilder supported advance research for hereditary ovarian cancer and the early detection of ovarian cancer. He did have some disagreements with the scientific community regarding mass screening for CA125, a plan which he promoted with no scientific support. In spite of all the research, ovarian cancer continues to be, to this day, as one of the most significant challenges, eluding early diagnosis and effective treatment. Ovarian cancer still claims many lives, but advances in research have helped to prolong life in many cases.

Gilda Radner died in 1989, about two years after her initial diagnosis. If she had lived without any ovarian cancer another decade or more, she would have been a candidate for genetic testing. If she was positive for the gene, it could have improved her odds of survival, by having a prophylactic surgery. Everyone should be grateful for her role in starting the public conversation by revealing her story and becoming the "face" of ovarian cancer.

Most ovarian cancers occur in post-menopausal women, and the incidence increases with age. 75 percent of ovarian cancers occur randomly with no inherited genes. Women are at higher risk for ovarian cancer if they are nulliparous, never on birth control pills, endometriosis, Menopause after age 50, have a family history of breast or ovarian cancer or test positive for BRCA or other implicated genes. Although it is rare to have ovarian cancer before age 40, when it happens earlier, it is very devastating and challenging, with the burden of making many decisions about the best treatments.

In 40 years, there have been significant improvements in the arena of ovarian cancer through the identification of high-risk patients and inherited genes. Tumor markers, though nonspecific, could be helpful in high-risk patients. Preventive therapy like birth control pills, prophylactic salpingectomy during a hysterectomy for benign conditions, and salpingo-oophorectomy in patients with a positive mutation for the BRCA gene have played a role in preventing or reducing the risk of ovarian cancer.

Women who have a family history of ovarian cancer should be advised to have genetic testing following the National Comprehensive Cancer Network (NCCN) guidelines (which change with updated research). Birth control pills reduce the risk of ovarian cancer by suppressing ovulation, and their prescription should be balanced with the other benefits and risks of usage. On the other hand, estrogen therapy for more than five years in postmenopausal women may slightly increase the risk of ovarian cancer. A woman is encouraged to seek care from her physician if she experiences two weeks of new-onset vague abdominal or pelvic pain, bloating or fullness of the abdomen, frequency of urination, or abnormal bleeding. In most cases, these symptoms are more often associated with benign etiology, but ovarian malignancy should be ruled out. Older women tend to seek care, while younger women tend to ignore these symptoms, thus delaying their diagnosis and possibly changing the probable outcomes.

Early diagnosis of ovarian cancer saves lives, but only 15% of ovarian cancers are diagnosed early because of the lack of proper screening methods. However, for high-risk patients with a family history of a first-degree relative with ovarian cancer or a positive BRCA gene, the CA125 blood test, a pelvic ultrasound, and a pelvic exam every six months are recommended. New research into liquid biopsy for early detection of cancers gives us hope for a very early diagnosis, which would save many lives from this devastating illness. Ovarian tumor diagnosed during a pelvic exam require a follow-up ultrasound to decipher the nature of the tumor and determine the need for surgery versus observation with a follow-up.

L.L's Story: Survival *and* Struggle

L.L was a 29-year-old single woman, who first came to see me in 1987 because of the abdominal discomfort with pain off and on for a couple of months. My exam revealed a large ovarian cyst. A pelvic ultrasound confirmed the diagnosis of the large complex ovarian cyst. I informed her that if she were older in her age, a malignancy would have been one of the possibilities, considering how complicated her cystic tumor was. I told her she still needed surgery, given the size and complexity of the cyst and her symptoms, it was most likely an endometrioma. I planned to remove the ovarian cyst only, with the possibility of removing the affected ovary but, reassured her she still would be able to get pregnant with the remaining fallopian tube and ovary. When I performed the surgery, I did have to remove the entire ovary. However, the final pathology results came back as invasive ovarian cancer, but the surface of the ovary was not involved.

I always dreaded notifying any patient or the family of a patient when the diagnosis was cancer, news that would change their lives forever. There are no words to express the burden of delivering the diagnosis to a 29-year-old and the devastating effect that it would have on her life. I discussed the diagnosis with a gynecologic oncologist who said one of the options was to remove the pelvic lymph nodes, the same side I removed the tumor, and to sample the other ovary. We advised her to get pregnant if she desired to have a baby, immediately after surgery. We recommended a hysterectomy along with the removal of both fallopian tubes and the other ovary, soon after the childbirth, to complete the treatment for her early ovarian cancer. The other option was to have a total hysterectomy and the removal of the fallopian tubes and the other ovary with lymph node dissection.

L.L decided to proceed with the conservative surgery option of unilateral lymph-node dissection and a sample of the other ovary. The oncologist performed her surgery with the lymph node dissection and a biopsy of the other ovary. The final pathology report of the second surgery was benign. She was in a long-term relationship with her boyfriend. She got engaged to be married and decided to get pregnant immediately. Fortunately, within a few months after the surgery, she became pregnant and delivered a healthy baby at full-term. A few months after childbirth, about a year and a half after I diagnosed her with ovarian cancer, L.L had a hysterectomy and a salpingo-oophorectomy, and the report no residual cancer.

L.L survived her cancer, and 30 years later, she is alive and doing well. Her initial response of joy and celebration surviving cancer was muted by the realization that she would never be able to have any more children. She also had to contend with the challenges of facing very early menopause with hot flashes, mood changes, insomnia, and vaginal atrophic changes. All these changes in her life created roller coast of emotions, which was a lifetime struggle of accepting what she lost in her quality of life. I know L.L never came to terms with her cancer and never stopped searching for answers as to why she had cancer at such a young age. I understood her emotional journey, but I did not have answers by which to give her the comfort she so wanted. After seeing her struggles and her quest to feel normal as a woman; I learned from L.L; cancer survival was not enough.

E.E's Story: Cancer and the Gift of Friendship

E.E was a 52-year-old married teacher with no children. I had immediately connected with her and she to me, maybe because neither of us had children. During her routine gynecology exam in 1988, I diagnosed E.E, who was menopausal, with a small mass on one of her ovaries. She had no symptoms of pain or bloating. As an appropriate follow-up, I ordered a pelvic ultrasound, which revealed a mildly complex cyst about three centimeters in size. The follow up of ovarian cysts, and the need for surgery depends on the age of the patient, the size of the cyst, and the nature and complexity of the cystic tumor. I informed her that the cyst was small and not very complicated, was most likely benign. However, in post menopause, ovaries rarely develop cysts in the absence of cyclical hormonal stimulation, and I would like to do a follow-up ultrasound in two months to ensure the stability of the cyst size and complexity of the cyst.

A repeat pelvic ultrasound, two months later, showed slight enlargement of the ovarian cyst to about four centimeters and that it had become more complex in nature. Considering her age and the complexity of the tumor, which was growing, I advised her to have surgery to rule out a malignancy even though it was most likely benign. I informed her I had no way of knowing whether it was benign or malignant without the surgery. She was somewhat surprised with my recommendation, was not ready to have the surgery, and wanted to get a second opinion, and I encouraged her to do so.

E.E called me back to let me know that the second opinion physician recommended observation with another follow-up ultrasound in two months. She said she was more confused now than ever, not knowing what to do. I scheduled an appointment to discuss this in person. During the visit, I talked to her and reiterated the reasons for surgery, considering her age, menopausal status, and the change in the size and complexity of the tumor in two months. I also said to her that a second opinion is just another opinion, not necessarily a better recommendation. She still needed to make the decision. I think she understood my reasoning and agreed to have surgery, which unfortunately revealed the diagnosis of ovarian cancer.

We both were thankful the cancer was stage 1, and the GYN oncologist suggested follow-up chemotherapy, which she received under his supervision. She was very positive and kept me abreast of her progress, always thanking me for my recommendation for her to have surgery. Two years went by, and she was doing well with no recurrence and still under the close surveillance of the gynecologic oncologist.

However, just two years after completing chemotherapy, she called me to let me know that her physician admitted her to the hospital for severe rectal bleeding. The tests revealed primary rectal cancer, not related to her ovarian cancer. Rectal cancer also has a significant mortality rate.

Subsequently, she spent the rest of her limited life in and out of the hospital, dealing with chemotherapy and its complications and the persistent disease. During one of her hospitalizations, I was walking in the hospital hallway when I saw her husband, and he let me know that E.E had been admitted to the hospital again and was dying. I went to visit her on Sunday morning, and we talked. She told me that she was ready to die and had accepted to undergo treatment one more time at the request of her husband, who was not prepared to let her go. I am not sure anyone ever accepts the death of a loved one, and most harbor the hope that the next treatment will be the one that will cure the disease, even when there is no hope. The acceptance of any illness is a journey for a patient's family as well as for the patient. E.E showed me the picture she chose to have over her casket and talked about the color of the dress she had picked out for her funeral. While I listened, I was amazed at her calm demeanor as she described her plans and wishes for her funeral.

During our conversation, an intern walked in to check on her. When he saw me in my lab coat talking to her, he was hesitant because he did not know who I was. She immediately introduced me to the intern as her friend who had come to visit her. I never forgot how she introduced me as a friend visiting her and then told him it was okay for him to come in and check on her. Did she know the impact the word "friend" had on me? What had I done to deserve receiving this gift of friendship from E.E? As she continued talking, I came to understand her to need to talk about her readiness for dying, her acceptance of death, and her choices for funeral arrangements. I had a hard time holding back my tears, but the only gift I could give her back was to listen. Then I hugged her, kissed her goodbye, knowing this was the last time I would ever see her.

After I left her room, I sobbed openly, walking down the floor hallway with no shame that somebody might be looking at me. E.E died within a couple of weeks while I was on vacation, and I was unable to attend her funeral. I was grateful that I had the opportunity to say my farewell. E.E did not win the battle against cancer but won the war by how she lived her life, spreading gifts of love and humanity. I lost a friend and will cherish her gift of friendship all my life.

Q.Q's Story: Severe Multiple Sclerosis, Cancer, and Decision-Making

In 2011, Q.Q was brought by wheelchair to my office by her husband. I had not seen Q.Q for more than twenty-five years since I had cared for her during three pregnancies and the delivery of her children. The last time I had seen her, she was in her thirties and perfect health. I was surprised to see her confined to a wheelchair, as she was just in her early 60s. Q.Q explained to me that she had been struggling with multiple sclerosis, which was diagnosed after her last child was born, and since then she had ignored the need to have any gynecology exams.

Q.Q came to see me because she was experiencing post-menopausal bleeding. At this point, Q.Q was immobile, and her husband was her primary caregiver. It was hard for me to see her in such a difficult condition. She said, despite her significant multiple sclerosis, she felt blessed to be able to share the joy of seeing her children grow up and looked at every day as a gift, rather than focusing on her limitations. Her visit was inspirational, not only because of her outlook on life but also because of her husband O.Q's dedication to her. O.Q was the primary caregiver for her including catheterization of her bladder, bathing, feeding, lifting, and keeping her clean. His situation could have been exhausting and one which might easily cause caregiver burnout. However, they seemed to have an excellent relationship with him joking "Thanks to Q.Q for being lightweight" as she weighed only around 90 pounds.

I explained to them the tests she needed for post-menopausal bleeding and left it up to Q.Q to decide if she wanted to proceed with the testing. She and her husband decided to go ahead with all the tests that I deemed necessary. I performed a uterine biopsy and ordered a pelvic ultrasound. Her uterine biopsy was normal. The ultrasound showed a four centimeter mildly complex cyst on one ovary. Her CA125 blood test was normal, though it is not the most reliable test with both a high false positive and a high false negative rate. However, in post-menopausal women, the CA125 is more reliable, and if it were elevated, I would have advised the surgery without any delay. I was concerned about doing surgery given her severe multiple sclerosis and the challenges it would bring with possible increased post-op complications that could even be life-threatening. I discussed the options of surgery versus observation with a follow-up ultrasound in two months and the benefits and risks of each option. I agreed with their decision to be watched, with a follow-up ultrasound in two months.

Q.Q's follow-up ultrasound four months later, showed the tumor to be more complex, and six centimeters in size. Her CT scan was normal other than confirming the diagnosis of a complex ovarian cyst. With the increase in size and complexity of the tumor, she needed surgery. I had a lengthy discussion with Q.Q and her husband about the possible diagnoses of benign, low-malignant, or malignant tumors. The conversation revolved mostly around what kind of surgery she would need, and how extensive the operation would be. If there was any possibility of malignancy on frozen section, I told her, it would prolong the length of surgery and possibly increase the risks from surgery due to her physical limitations and low BMI. Ambulation after surgery is one of the most crucial post-op activities that one would need to reduce the risk of blood clots in legs and lungs. We talked about the recommended operation being a hysterectomy (removal of the uterus), bilateral salpingo-oophorectomy (removal of tubes and ovaries), excision of the lymph nodes and an omentectomy (removal of a layer of fat inside the abdomen) to assess the stage and spread of the disease. Tumors can spread microscopically, and it can be difficult to determine the spread of cancer unless a pathologist looks at it under a microscope.

I explained that Q.Q would benefit from minimally invasive surgery, causing less pain and allowing her to increase her mobility more quickly with daily passive bike exercise. I told her that I could start with the robot-assisted laparoscopy surgery to remove the affected tube and ovary, and would send the specimen for a frozen section (preliminary testing). If pathology showed malignancy, I would need to perform a laparotomy with a big incision in the abdomen to perform total omentectomy along with the lymph node dissection. There was no guarantee she would survive such extensive surgery. I also informed her that she would need chemotherapy if there were a diagnosis of malignancy. Q.Q, with her husband's support, decided to go ahead with robot-assisted laparoscopy for salpingo-oophorectomy. However, if the frozen section showed pre-malignancy or malignancy, she decided to have a hysterectomy and salpingo-oophorectomy of the other ovary, but most likely not the more extensive surgery recommended. In case she changed her mind, I decided to have the gynecologic oncologist on standby, to perform the more extensive operation

After our discussion, I had grave concerns in my mind about her surgical outcomes. Would she be able to tolerate extensive surgery to determine the stage of cancer and would she survive chemotherapy, given her neurological disease and low BMI?

I performed Q.Q's surgery on Jan 3rd, 2012, confirming a six-centimeter cyst, but with no other visible lesions. However, the frozen section showed ovarian malignancy. Usually, in such cases, a gynecologic oncologist would perform a laparotomy with a large incision to have better access to remove the omentum (layer of fat) and lymph nodes. I informed her husband and her grown children of the dilemma at hand. I suggested to them that I could perform a complete hysterectomy and remove the other fallopian tube and ovary. Because of our earlier discussion, we knew Q.Q might not have wanted any further treatment beyond hysterectomy and salpingo-oophorectomy, and her husband and family agreed with this decision. It was one of the most difficult professional decisions I ever had to make because there was no perfect answer, but I leaned toward giving her the best quality of life she could enjoy. I also informed my gynecologic oncologist, who had been on standby, about the decision not to perform extensive surgery for evaluation of the stage of the disease. I completed the rest of the surgery.

Her recovery from minimally invasive surgery was slow as expected, but her spirit and her determination to recover was never in question. The uterus and her other tube and ovary were benign, but fluid washings showed a few atypical cells, suggesting she had either stage 1C ovarian cancer or benign reactive cells. It was difficult to know the stage of her disease because of the incomplete surgery performed. However, because of the positive atypical cells, she was a candidate for chemotherapy. Q.Q and her husband were acutely aware of the nature of malignancy and that the surgery was incomplete for staging and not having chemotherapy would increase her risk for recurrence and eventually might take her life. Nonetheless, she declined chemotherapy. I advised her to get a second opinion with a gynecologic oncologist. They decided to see a gynecologic oncologist at the University of Michigan for a second opinion. After much discussion, considering her physical condition and the risks of chemotherapy, Q.Q decided against chemotherapy.

Q.Q told me we are like "soul sisters," and she felt I knew what she wanted and how far she wanted to go with the surgery. Q.Q and O.Q are highly educated and understood the implications of their decisions. She made me feel better, though, I knew there was no perfect answer in this very complicated situation. I wish I had had a crystal ball to know what the best treatment for her was, without increasing her risks and making her quality of life any worse. There are many occasions, where the physician is called on to make a judgment call by paying attention to the whole person, rather than following the usual standards of care. It was one of those occasions over which I lost sleep, wondering if I had helped her or hurt her.

In January 2018, Q.Q and O.Q called me for advice for one of their family members and informed me that she is cancer-free, six years after her surgery. I was deeply touched to hear from them and was pleased to know that she is doing well. Despite the challenges in their lives, I was happy to see that Q.Q and her husband, enjoying their children and grandchildren and found joy in all that life has to offer. Being a witness, to how Q.Q decided to live her life with the love and support of her husband and the family, focusing on positive experiences, and emotionally overcoming her physical limitations has been an inspiration to me.

K.K's Story: A Struggle with the Risk and an Understanding of the BRCA Gene

In the 1980s, a family registry for ovarian cancer was started to identify patients at high risk of developing ovarian cancer. A decade or so later, the genetic research identified the genes BRCA1 and BRCA2 linked to a higher risk of developing both breast and ovarian cancer. The women who have carcinomas of the breast and ovaries from *inherited* genes are about 10-15%. However, if women carry a mutation of BRCA1 or BRCA2, the risk of having malignancy is very high (for breast cancer, 70 to 80%; for ovarian cancer, 20% to 45%). Prophylactic mastectomy and salpingo-oophorectomy reduce the risks of the breast and ovarian cancer by 90%.

After 2001, according to the NCCN guidelines for breast and ovarian cancers, every patient in my practice was assessed for risk factors. I counseled any patient who was at risk to have the inherited gene and discussed the potential benefit of genetic screening and the potential risk of breast and ovarian cancer. It was incredibly confusing to my patients that they could be carrying a gene, which could result in cancer when they felt healthy and normal. When a family member is positive for a BRCA gene, every family member needs to get tested per NCCN guidelines. If she/he is negative for the inherited gene, their children would be negative. It becomes a different challenge when the family member is reluctant to be tested, creating conflicts and hurt feelings among the family members. These are highly charged emotional issues. You cannot blame anyone for the decisions they make; ultimately, it is an individual journey.

Patients who understood the explanation still had concerns: if they were positive for one of the genes, could they be denied health insurance coverage and life insurance coverage for a pre-existing condition? In the early days, many, if not all, insurance policies did not cover the cost of the test, which was very expensive. Until the Affordable Care Act of 2010, such a pre-existing condition proved to be a big challenge for many of my patients to overcome even when they decided to have the test. I had written many letters to insurance companies explaining the benefits of having the test and the risks of not having the test.

There are many challenges in deciding to have the test: the first being the patient's acceptance of the risk and the fear of knowing the results that could change not only their life but their children's lives too. (There is a 50% chance of inheriting the gene if a family member is positive.) Then there is the added burden of deciding an optimal time to have the test, before or after childbearing. Also, women have to choose whether to have surgery or close surveillance with testing every six months while also dealing with the ultimate challenge of health insurance coverage. I realized often; it is tough for many patients to decide to have the test, especially if they are normal and their parents had no cancer. About 20% of the women positive for the BRCA gene never develop breast cancer, and about 50% to 60% never develop ovarian cancer. Sometimes it takes many years of counseling before a woman decides to undergo the test.

K.K, in her mid-40s, had been seeing me for a few years for routine gynecology exams. After reviewing her strong family history of premenopausal breast cancer on her maternal side, I counseled her about the risks of the inherited BRCA genes. Her mother was at high risk for the inherited gene, which in turn meant that if she were positive, there would be a 50% chance of K.K and her siblings carrying the gene. Her mother was in her 70s and had no history of breast or ovarian cancer. Every year at her annual exam, I would again discuss the need for genetic testing of her mother. After a few years, to my surprise, she did take her mother for genetic screening, and the result was positive for the BRCA1 gene. None of the children wanted to believe the test and, instead, wanted to repeat their mother's test. Genetic counselors advised them otherwise, and ultimately, all the children decided to have the test done. In this family of four children, all of them were positive for the gene. Out of all the families of my patients whom I tested, this family was the only one where everyone was positive for the inherited gene. K.K, who was the youngest in the family, was genuinely shocked by the results, as, so far, none of her family members had cancers linked to the inherited gene.

K.K made an appointment to discuss her results and receive counseling with her husband present. I talked to her about the risks of developing breast and ovarian cancer. For the breast cancer risk, I discussed the benefits and risks of monitoring with mammograms, breast ultrasounds, and breast MRIs versus a prophylactic bilateral mastectomy.

On the other hand, for ovarian cancer, the tests for monitoring and early diagnosis have both high false positive and high false negative rates, making it difficult to monitor successfully. The prophylactic removal of both ovaries and fallopian tubes will reduce the risk by over 90%. Even after the procedure, there was a future risk of peritoneal carcinomatosis, cancer of the lining of the abdomen. During the development of the embryo, the peritoneal lining shares a cell lining with the ovaries. Another potential future risk factor will be if a small portion of the fallopian tube, at the junction of the uterus surrounded by uterine musculature, may not be entirely excised during the bilateral salpingo-oophorectomy. To minimize the risk further, I also advised a hysterectomy to reduce the risk further. Performing a hysterectomy was not a recommended guideline, but I started with this recommendation after a patient of mine who was positive for the BRCA1 gene and had undergone bilateral salpingo-oophorectomy developed a papillary serous carcinoma of the uterus, which was similar to ovarian cancer.

I discussed with K.K the benefits and risks of surgery. She and her husband listened to my recommendations, and she said she needed time to think about my suggestions for operation. She was 48 at the time, and her mammogram, MRI, and ultrasound of her breasts were normal, so were the CA125 and CEA blood tests and the pelvic ultrasound to monitor her ovaries.

I did not hear from K.K for about three months. One day, without an appointment, she walked into my office with tears in her eyes and told my staff she wanted to have surgery immediately. They gave her an appointment for a surgical consult the same week. During my consult with her, she shared how devastated she was to have learned that one of her sisters who lived in California had just been diagnosed with Stage 3 ovarian cancer, while she had been deciding what to do after she was tested positive for the BRCA gene. I performed K.K's surgery within the next couple of weeks. She had Stage 3 endometriosis, but no cancer.

K.K stated, she felt she had time; after all, her mother had never developed cancer, so K.K thought she would not either. It is typical for most of us to respond to our own experiences. The risk she was taking became real to her only when her sister developed ovarian cancer. I have seen other women react in the same manner as K.K did in the absence of a personal/family history of cancer. Our intellectual understanding of the facts is so far removed from our emotional responses, even when we are at risk of developing deadly malignancies. As a physician, I could only hope that any patient who is at risk but had decided against the testing or surgical treatment would not have to face a situation like K.K's sister did. It takes time to come to terms with this burdensome inheritance and decide on the treatment choices available to them.

X.X's Story: Uterine Cancer and Advanced Medical Directives

Uterine cancer is the fourth most common cancer in women. Every year over 50,000 women are diagnosed with the most common form of uterine cancer—adenocarcinoma of endometrium—and about 9,000 women die from it. In most cases, endometrial cancer is diagnosed early, and at Stage 1, the five-year cure rate is about 90%. The average age of a woman diagnosed with endometrial cancer is 60. Women who have endometrial cancer in pre-menopausal years should be checked for an inherited gene for Lynch Syndrome which is also linked to colon cancer, to a lesser extent, ovarian cancer, and few other cancers. The risk factors that increase endometrial cancer are age, nulliparity (bore no children), obesity, estrogen hormone therapy, Tamoxifen (a drug for breast cancer prevention), women with anovulatory (infrequent) periods, a strong family history of colon cancer at a younger age or a family history of premenopausal endometrial cancer.

Any post-menopausal women with even one episode of spotting should be evaluated by an endometrial biopsy and an ultrasound of the pelvis. If both tests are normal, the patient should be observed but will need a D&C if she has any further episode of spotting or bleeding. It is equally important to evaluate patients in the perimenopausal phase with prolonged or frequent periods. Abnormal periods are typical in the premenopausal stage, but other pathology, including pre-malignancy or malignancy, should be ruled out. Once diagnosed with a malignancy, staging surgery should be performed, along with the hysterectomy, removal of both tubes and ovaries, as well as lymph node dissection. The stage of the disease is determined by the evaluation of the size and depth of the tumor and the status of lymph-node involvement or involvement of the other organs. The prognosis and treatment depend upon the grade of cancer as well as the stage of cancer. Follow-up treatment with local radiation and chemotherapy also depends on the stage and grade of the disease.

X.X was an 87-year-old woman who had been my patient for several years when she made an appointment to see me for evaluation of a single episode of spotting. X.X led a very active life, was independent and the caregiver for her 92-year-old husband. Serving as a caregiver was not an unusual situation in aging female population. I explained to her that the most common causes of post-menopausal spotting are benign, but malignancy must always be ruled out. To rule out malignancy, I needed to do a uterine biopsy and a pelvic ultrasound, if she chose for me to proceed. When a patient is in her late 80s, what is the morally correct approach for evaluation and treatment, given this limited longevity of life? How aggressive should one be? My recommendations for an active, very healthy woman might be different than for someone who is suffering from multiple comorbid conditions in poor physical health with the limited longevity of life. I gave all my patients options, for both testing and treatment, and then helped them make their decisions with their family members.

X.X said she wanted to have a biopsy and ultrasound performed to have the information but jokingly told me not to find any cancer. She expressed the fear of ending up in a nursing home like her 95-year-old sister. It is every person's worst fear: ending up in a nursing home and wishing she/he could die in their own home. I went ahead with the biopsy, and the diagnosis came back as endometrial cancer. I performed D&C to provide a further evaluation. The report showed Grade 1 endometrial cancer. Her pelvic ultrasound showed an enlarged multi-cystic ovary. I had a lengthy discussion with her, in the presence of her daughters, about the known diagnosis of endometrial cancer and the unknown status of her enlarged ovary with possible malignancy. I explained surgical options to X.X including surgical staging and possible follow-up chemotherapy, which would depend on the diagnosis and the stage of the disease.

After much discussion of the benefits and risks, she decided not to have surgery. I explained to her we would not be able to know cancer's pace of progression, and that while she might die from other causes, it was possible if cancer progressed quickly enough, she might die from the disease. She accepted my recommendation of treatment with 80 milligrams a day of Megace to suppress her endometrial cancer, and I advised her to call me if she experienced abdominal bloating, pain, persistent bleeding, or changes in bowel habits. Otherwise, we would continue the medication with no further evaluation, but I would see her every six months, to make sure she was not experiencing any new symptoms.

X.X continued to lead an active life, caring for her husband, who died about a year and a half later. After her husband died, she visited Florida for six months. When she returned, two years after her initial diagnosis, she came to see me, just before I retired. She had continued to do well on Megace, and recently I was told she is doing well, that is four years after her initial diagnosis of endometrial cancer. In X.X's case, advanced medical directives with clear direction from her helped me and her family to prescribe the treatment of her choice, not what we would have done if she was not an active participant and did not have advanced medical directives. It was a perfect example why everyone needs to have an advance medical directive.

My Family's Story: A Story of Cancer Too Close to Home

In 2013, my own family had to face the emotional toll of a cancer diagnosis. My younger sister called me on the morning of July 2nd from India. The conversation that ensued still seems surreal to me. My brother-in-law had had a colonoscopy, and his physician diagnosed him with a large tumor in the sigmoid colon, which was confirmed by a CT scan. They were waiting for the biopsy report.

The biopsy confirmed the diagnosis of malignancy. Most people think it is never going to happen to them or their family until it happens. We were no different, and I was no different. After the initial shock of the news wore off, my primary role was to give my sister and her husband support and reassurance, to provide them with a sense of security that we were all in this together. While it was hard to imagine what they were going through, I tried to reassure my sister over the phone, that my brother-in-law would be okay. While attempting to encircle them with love and support to make them feel we had their back, I felt utterly helpless because I could not be there with them in person.

There was not enough time for us to go through the whole gamut of emotions. We had to focus on the treatment, and whether my brother-in-law should have the surgery done in India or the U.S. With the consensus of my two nieces, who live in the U.S., I decided he should have his surgery at Providence Hospital. I talked to Dr. Ernie Drelichman, a colorectal surgeon, who was very generous in reviewing my brother-in-law's tests and agreed to perform surgery. I will be forever grateful for all his generosity and support through the entire process. I made financial arrangements with the Hospital CEO and CFO. My sister and brother-in-law flew in from India, and my brother-in-law's surgery was scheduled a week later. The whole week was busy with getting the necessary tests done. My brother-in-law was strong and never expressed his emotions. My sister, who is usually very emotional, was holding up well until the two days before her husband's surgery.

Two days before surgery, she pretty much fell apart, worried about the diagnosis, possible stage of cancer, and what might come after. She was unable to sleep, and she expressed that she felt her head was going to split open. I wanted to take her pain away and give her the guarantee that all would be well. I kept reminding myself of all the cancer survivors I had encountered and tried to reassure the family and my self with the "mantra" that colon cancers have a good prognosis and let us take one step at a time. I was worried that my sister would not be able to make it to the hospital the day of surgery to support her husband, and I could not imagine my brother-in-law going in for surgery without having his wife there.

Everything felt like it was happening in slow motion with me at the center, making all the decisions and giving the support to all the family, while trying not to fall apart myself. Their two daughters came in the evening before surgery. My sister drew strength from all of us and made it to the hospital, to be with her husband before surgery. Dr. Drelichman performed the surgery without any glitches, and my brother-in-law was phenomenal in how well he handled the operation. He was a very motivated patient; he recovered very quickly. He was very inspirational to all of us. All the gestures of love and support that my family and I received during visits by CEO Dr. Wiemann, pathologist, Dr.Barry Hershman, the nursing staff, the nursing directors, and all the ancillary support personnel during his hospitalization touched me deeply.

His final diagnosis was rectosigmoid cancer with optimal surgical resection of the sigmoid colon and the removal of more than the required number of lymph nodes.

The genetic testing for Lynch syndrome was negative. We were thankful to Dr. Ernie Drelichman for his expertise, so my brother-in-law would have a better chance of survival. After much discussion, he was advised to have chemotherapy. My sister and brother-in-law went back to India to receive chemotherapy.

When he was in the final month of completing the six months of chemotherapy, my sister, his wife, was diagnosed with breast cancer on a routine mammogram. My sister dealt with her cancer with strength and hope and had a lumpectomy followed by radiation therapy. Her breast cancer was Stage 1 and Grade 1, her lymph node sampling was negative. My friend Ramana, a pathologist, helped me get oncogene typing done, and we were relieved to know that the test results showed low risk for a recurrence and she did not need chemotherapy. However, I was worried about her emotional state. Although she was trying to be strong outwardly, I felt guilty for not being there for her to give the words of support and comfort she needed.

No matter what the stage of the cancer is, any diagnosis involving the word "cancer" raises one's level of fear and anxiety. A cancer patient needs support, strength, and love from one's spouse. The worst part of my sister and her husband's situation was that they both were diagnosed with cancer only six months apart. As they were each trying to deal with the emotions of having been diagnosed with cancer in such a short interval, I wondered how hard it must have been for them to support one another. Four and half years later, both are cancer-free. Every time they go for follow-up tests, I feel their concern about the possible news the testing might bring, even though I firmly believe they have an excellent chance of staying cancer-free.

It is difficult to express how inadequate I felt and still feel in helping my sister and her husband's cancer journey. I would indeed like to understand their inner conflicts and fears and walk with them on their journey, as they find a path in coming to terms with cancer, and move forward in life.

During all the years, I have seen patients with cancer, most survived, but some did not. I learned more about individuals and their journeys than cancer itself, and they left an indelible impression on me. I often think about; V.W's fear of having cancer leading to her death, and my limitation in saving her life; N.N's fight to survive to see her children grow up, and me thinking about what-ifs; F.F's courage and pragmatic approach to life and death; H.H and K.K's resilience in their struggle with the burden of carrying genes; L.L's journey of cancer survival and struggles with the quality of life; Q.Q's quiet strength and the dignity in dealing with two serious illnesses; X.X's pragmatic approach toward life and cancer; and E.E's generosity and the gift of friendship while she was dying.

In the past 38 years, during my practice, medical science has made some progress in the diagnosis and the understanding and the treatment of all cancers, more significantly in some, not so much in others. What gives me hope and optimism is that we are on the verge of making great strides in fighting one of the most devastating illnesses facing humanity. It is the improvement in prevention and screening of cancers which increases the chances of survival in some and prolongs longevity in others. There is a good chance for better outcomes, with the advances in understanding tumor genetics and inherited genes, new diagnostic tools like liquid biopsy, and new treatments based on gene mutation. The science of medicine is an arc that bends slowly, it is true, but always is making progress, however, slow it may feel when you are in the middle of the storm of experiencing pain and suffering. It is not so different a paradigm than what President Obama would say about the arc of history.

Later Years of My Practice, 2003-2016

Hope is being able to see that there is light,
despite all the darkness.
--- Desmond Tutu

In 2003, the same year that my mother died, I ventured into a new phase of my life. I started my solo practice and went back to my roots of patient-centered care, with highly professional and supportive staff. No longer did patients experience voice prompted responses when they called. The team answered all the calls. Patients received the service that they deserved with a dedicated nurse triaging all my patients' medical calls. As the focus of my practice had been gynecology since 1999, I was involved in serving the women by meeting their needs in all aspects of their health. In previous chapters, I have addressed my role as a gynecologist in caring for my patients during menopause, surgeries, cancer diagnosis and treatment. I was inspired every day, listening to "my patients' day-to-day challenges" of living life. Many of them faced the issues of divorce, raised children as single mothers, struggled to understand the sexuality of their children, cared for their children with cancer, mental illness, drug abuse, and supported their older parents with dementia, or living with the burdens aging.

Depression and eating disorders are two common disorders that many teenagers, as well as women, face. Depression can be related to biochemical imbalances, in which case it leads to a lifetime of struggle, requiring a lifetime of treatment. Depression may also be situational, in response to life-altering events like divorce, illness, or the death of a loved one, which can be helped by counseling and possibly a short treatment period of medication. Eating disorders, on the other hand, are even more challenging than depression as there are no proper treatments for eating disorders, and they often result in a struggle throughout life.

D.L's Story: Grit and the Power of Love Overcomes Anorexia

D.L was 19 years old, young, and pretty with very long hair all the way down to her waist. She was engaged to be married when she came to see me for her first gynecology exam. She was full of energy with a beautiful smile on her face and radiated charm with a childlike innocence when she talked and shared her excitement about her marriage to her fiancé in the next few months. After getting married, she had two girls within the next few years. Later, she expressed to me the difficulties of her marriage. She told me that she was in a verbally abusive relationship and stated she had been sexually abused as a child by an immediate member of her family.

After counseling, she ultimately initiated a divorce from her husband. Around the same time, she confronted her family member about the sexual abuse she had to endure as a child. As a result, her relationship with her family severed. Her family of origin was a well-respected middle-class family, and her family members denied her allegation. She felt isolated and like no one had her back. Her older daughter became estranged from her and decided to live with her ex-husband. It was an intensely contested divorce, and the father used the children as pawns, giving them what they wanted and blaming D.L for all that was happening in their daughters' lives. D.L shared her perspective with me about what was going on in her life, and although I had no way of confirming it, I did notice that she appeared to be spiraling down into depression. Every time I saw her during this crisis, she did not seem to be getting any better and also had begun and continued to lose a significant amount of weight. She was diagnosed with an eating disorder, anorexia nervosa.

Above all, D.L loved her children, and she was emotionally drained and grieved about having lost the contact with her older daughter. She was hospitalized several times a year to treat different conditions because, as a result of anorexia, her cardiovascular system and kidneys were damaged. Given her significant mental and physical difficulties, I was not sure if she would survive and make it through her next hospital admission. Nonetheless, while she was getting help with these significant life-threatening challenges, she never stopped fighting to be better and accepted all the treatments for the considerable afflictions of depression, anorexia, and the other resulting physical ailments. Through several years of this struggle with anorexia, depression, and physical limitations, she never lost the sparkle in her eye, the beautiful smile on her face, or her childlike innocence when she talked, all of which reminded me of her first visit with me when she was 19.

During this time, an incredible change happened in her life that helped her to love herself again. She found love, a man who loved her for all that she was. They got married and have been married for more than two decades now. Her second husband certainly has her back and has been standing by her side, through thick and thin. As time passed, I saw changes as she came to terms with her past and accepted the lack of relationship with her older daughter. She gained weight and her physical condition stabilized. Her younger daughter was doing well and thriving under her care. She learned her older daughter had had a baby, and while she felt sad, she did not go back down through that spiral of depression. Her second daughter became a nurse, got married, and had a baby. D.L was able to connect with her older daughter again and has been able to see her other grandchildren. Additionally, she developed some communication with her parents.

Today, D.L is in her 50s, walks with a cane, and is on multiple medications. However, I see that she is happy with her life, which includes a loving husband, her grown-up daughters, and grandchildren. She is not only living; she is loving life encircled by the love of her family. After thirty-plus years, she did not lose the beautiful smile or her childlike innocence. The day before I retired, she brought me a series of pictures, some from when she was young, pregnant and with her newborn babies and others of her daughters with their babies. She also brought me a bracelet of teal crystal beads with a note saying that teal stands for: green for growth, strength, and spirit and blue for calm, gentle, serene feelings. Her card also said that for her the color teal reflects women and women's health.

D.L, now in her fifties, displayed grit, strength, love, and determination, even while fighting for her life in the face of death. During the most challenging years of her life dealing with depression and anorexia, I was relieved to see her at each of her visits, to know she had survived another year. She visited the deepest holes of darkness and was able to draw herself back up into the light of life. Like the color of teal, she represents growth, strength, spirit, calmness, and a gentle serenity, while going through the storms of life. D.L is a real winner.

C.C and Her Son's Story: The Importance of Hope "Against All Odds"

I have seen many mothers when faced with an illness of one of their children, immediately spring into action, even when the medical community gives them a message of no hope. Such mothers would go to the ends of the earth to find a treatment to help their children recover while going through immense fear and grief, not knowing what the future holds. Most mothers are natural nurturers and have a "protection gene" when it comes to their children, much as a tigress does in protecting her cubs when there is looming danger.

C.C had seen me for many years for gynecology care. During one of her visits, she talked to me about her son, who was involved in a major accident, who was in early 20's. One summer evening, when her son had been driving home from Canada, the sun was glaring in his eyes, and he did not see the eighteen-wheeler. His car crashed into the truck so hard that it went right underneath it. After being rescued, EMT took C.C's son to the closest hospital. He was in a coma, the medical team initiated the required supportive treatment, and his parents were informed. Fortunately, they lived only a couple of hours away and immediately went to be with their son. None of us could imagine the fear and anxiety that C.C and her husband experienced, seeing their 20-year-old son in a coma and not knowing if he would ever survive or if he recovered what he would be. Physicians told C.C and her husband that their son's brain was swelling (cerebral edema), which could be lethal if the swelling did not respond to the standard treatment.

C.C, though not in the medical field, was aware of partial craniectomy—removal of part of the cranial bone or otherwise known as skullcap—to relieve the pressure from rapid swelling on the vital areas of the brain. The Canadian physicians told the parents they would not be able to perform the procedure. Physicians also said to the parents, most likely that their son would end up in a permanent vegetative state. C.C refused to accept—as many mothers would in a similar situation—that her son would never recover from the coma and decided to have him transferred to one of the best medical institutions in the Detroit area. There, they performed a decompressive partial craniectomy to allow his brain to swell and to decrease the compression effects on the vital areas of his brain. As he continued to be in a coma during the first few weeks, physicians at the reputable hospital also told her that he would most likely end up in a permanent vegetative state.

As he slowly recovered from his acute brain injury, he recovered from the coma beyond the expectations of the physicians who were caring for him during his hospitalization and inpatient rehabilitation. Once they released from the inpatient rehab, the arduous journey of long-term rehabilitation and recovery started for C.C's son. It was a new journey, not only for C.C's son but also for his parents and his younger brother, eight years' junior to him. He had a significant closed head injury with amnesia as well as weakness on one half of his body. C.C dedicated her life to her son's recovery in every which way she could help him. C.C's son had been a music student, and she included music therapy as part of his rehab. Though she tried to do her best for her younger son during this time, she could not help but see that her younger son felt ignored and expressed jealousy about his older brother getting the most attention, even wishing to be in his brother's place.

C.C is a strong woman and managed to help her younger son by involving him in his older brother's recovery. Every year when she came to see me, we talked about her son and his progress. Two years after the accident, she was very excited to let me know that her son was able to slightly move one of his fingers on the side of his body that had been affected. He continued to make progress over the years. Only families of the victims of acute brain injury understand the joys of any improvement, no matter how little the change may be in our eyes, giving them the hope for the future.

We have learned more about the role of music therapy in healing and repairing networks connecting neurons. Music is being used with wounded veterans and was used to aid the recovery of Gabby Gifford, the congresswoman who was the victim of a gunshot wound to the brain. I have always wondered what would have been the outcome for C.C's son, if C.C, under the most extraordinarily stressful conditions did not take the prompt actions with her son lingering between life and death. Would he have suffered a life of permanent disability, if his parents did not decide to transfer him to another institution? What would have been the outcome, if he had not had the decompression craniectomy to reduce the devastating effects of cerebral edema? How much of his background as a musician and C.C's initiation of the music therapy played a role in his profound recovery? C.C's love for her son, her ability to think quickly on her feet, and music therapy, as well as her son's courage and perseverance most likely helped in his recovery.

As a human being, not as a physician, I am inspired to see how a mother fights to protect her children—especially when they are pushed into a corner by the direst situation— and makes a difference. Many mothers seem to be able to reach down into their inner core to find the courage and rise above their fear and despair to deal with the situation at hand. Mothers with a can-do attitude, and with an unwavering mindset, as strong as steel, they find ways to save their children from death or disability. In C.C's situation, she saved her son's future by questioning the medical profession and demanding the best available option, which resulted in the correct course of treatment.

It is easy to understand how a mother would react with denial when she receives such traumatic news. Some never accept that their child will never recover, even after many years without progress. When is the right time to tell the parents that there is no hope of recovery? As C.C's son was young and had no underlying disease, was it too early for his parents to receive such a bleak prognosis? I encouraged C.C to write a letter to her son's physicians about her son's incredible progress so that they might get some insight into such a situation for future reference.

During her last visit before my retirement, C.C told me her son can walk with a cane, had graduated from college, and has a girlfriend. He is even planning to move to Colorado where his girlfriend lives. C.C was happy that her son was trying to move on with his life. It was such a giant leap forward from the day of the accident, with an unknown future to a future full of anticipation and hope. At the same time, C.C was also apprehensive and anxious, wondering if he would be able to spread his wings and fly on his own into the winds of life without falling. C.C was just like a mother bird, watching her fledgling as he prepares to fly for the first time, leaving the nest that the mother built to protect him from harm. It was my privilege to know C.C and her story of a mother's love, a son's courage, and a family's perseverance.

J.J's Story: An Amazing Woman, A Hero

Physical disability changes the life of any person, forever presenting the struggle to manage day-to-day chores with dignity and to not give into the hopelessness that one might feel when one cannot function like everyone else. It is difficult for anyone at any age when faced with a physical limitation. It is harder to imagine what it was like for a young child, who was physically active one day and unable to move the next day, due to an accident and the confusion and the fear that goes with the tragedy.

J.J was in her early 20's when she started seeing me as a patient. When J.J came in her wheelchair, I did not see a wheelchair; I just saw J.J She was confident, with a smile that lit up the room, making everyone around her feel comfortable and giving the impression that there was nothing she could not do. I just loved seeing her. When I took her history, I learned that when she was 11 years old, she had been in a major accident that killed her father and severed her spinal cord, leaving her paraplegic. What her mother had to go through is beyond what any one of us dare to understand, to be strong for her daughter who was frightened and confused, not knowing what is happening to her, while grieving for the loss of her husband.

Once J.J recovered from the acute phase of the accident, everyone around her concentrated on making her stronger both physically and emotionally, so she could be as self-reliant as possible. One of her physical therapists—who happened to be another patient of mine—became her lifetime friend. She had a phenomenal attitude toward life, and I wondered what made her who she is today? Could it be due to her mother's dedication and love, J.J's survival instinct, and strength, or the commitment of her dedicated medical staff? Most likely all of the above. She was physically so strong that she was able to get on the examination table without any help, by using just her upper body. She had a great personality and a friendly nature and never considered herself as limited, either in her mind or spirit. She dealt with her inability to walk and the need for daily self-catheterization of the bladder multiple times as part of her routine life. Her mother seemed to have done such a fabulous job instilling confidence in her at that young age that she is not defined by her paralyzed legs, but by who she is as a person.

I was not surprised at all when she told me a wonderful man had fallen in love with her, and they were engaged to be married. It brought tears to my eyes; when I saw the sparks in her eyes and the big beautiful grin on her face, when she spoke about her fiancé. What a lovely man he had to be to see her for who she was and to fall in love with this beautiful, inspirational person! Just before her wedding, she came to see me, and for the first time, she expressed self-doubt and anxiety about going down the aisle in a wheelchair. We talked, and I validated her fears as being normal, but reassured her that no one was going to see her wheelchair, but instead would see the beautiful person she indeed was inside and out. I advised her to enjoy this extraordinary day in her life of getting married to this exceptional man. Later she told me she had had a beautiful day and her mother walked her down the aisle. What a great moment for both of them!

When the time came to decide to start a family, unlike many women, she expressed her worries about how she would be as a mom, given her disability. Would she be able to meet the physical needs of her children and would pregnancy increase her risks of blood clots in her legs and lungs because of her immobility? After much discussion, she decided to become pregnant, which unfortunately led to a miscarriage. After that painful experience, she and her husband decided to look at alternatives.

J.J and her husband decided to attempt surrogacy. Through this procedure, they had twins who are thriving and seem to be doing very well. J.J settled into the motherhood with great joy and confidence with her husband standing right by her side. At every visit, J.J shared with me her children's activities and their progress with a huge smile, which exuded the joy of being a mother.

This young lady, at age 11, had lost both her father and the function of her legs on the same day. Within a matter of a few seconds, her life changed forever. She accepted and adapted to her new life with courage, with a can-do attitude and a spirit that brings a smile to the faces of people around her. It has been an astounding experience for me to witness J.J full of love and effervescence, not harboring any bitterness and I truly cherished the joy of being her physician. When I think about her, a smile comes to my face, and I do not feel any sadness, knowing her life is full. I have visual images of J.J, with her incredible loving husband by her side, watching their two children grow up in a house full of love and happiness. I used to tell J.J that she is my hero, and I meant it.

D.V's Story: The Complexities of Mental Illness

Depression does not afflict a particular race, ethnicity, economic class, or family background. Most family members respond to this challenge with disbelief, shame, and confusion, wondering how it could be possible one of their loved ones is suffering from depression. I see mothers struggling with their children's depression and personality disorders, not knowing how to help their children and being scared every day, wondering if this is the day they are going to hear the child has ended his/her life or has even become homicidal.

Mental illness is one of life's most challenging events, and the health care system denies many patients and their families the care they deserve, as well as sufficient guidelines and a support system. For many years, people who have mental illness were looked down upon—even by their families and the patients themselves—as having an overblown condition that society perceives as a sign of weakness rather than illness. Even discussing mental illness was taboo, and for families there are no useful resources from which to draw upon, to understand what their family member was experiencing. Signs and symptoms of Mental illness are the changes in mood, behavior, and the presence of hallucinations or delusions. Most of the affected families do not possess an understanding of all the intricacies of the brain's chemical malfunction. Such chemical malfunction may lead to many of the most complicated and misunderstood illnesses, which may be genetically linked and afflict many generations in one family.

D.V was in her late twenties when she came to see me as a patient. She had one child and was having difficulty getting pregnant a second time. After an appropriate workup, I diagnosed her with endometriosis. She never did get pregnant again and was very upset about it. She appeared to be unable to get over the grief and felt a loss of support from her husband, whether it was real or perceived. A few years after our first encounter, I performed a hysterectomy and bilateral salpingo-oophorectomy because of the worsening symptoms of endometriosis, unresponsive to medical treatment and were significantly affecting her quality of life. After the hysterectomy, she had to come to terms with the fact that it forever shut the door to have any more children. D.V, who had been depressed already, was thrown over the edge into severe depression, resulting in many suicide attempts and subsequent hospitalizations. Fortunately, she had a great relationship with her psychiatrist, who helped her through many suicide attempts, trips in and out of the hospitals, and changes in medications over many years.

After many years of struggle, her physician decided she would be a candidate for electroconvulsive therapy (ECT). After ECT, her life stabilized with the help of medications. I could see a change in her, where she appeared to have found peace in her soul. She started enjoying the relationship with her husband, who had stood by her during the severest symptoms of her mental illness.

During the most challenging years of her mental illness, D.V would tell me that her relationship with her only child, a daughter, was distant and remote. Her husband was the primary nurturer and provider for their daughter, and it only made the situation worse for D.V I always wondered what had thrown her into depression; she had seemed normal until she had difficulty having the second baby. If she did not need the hysterectomy and bilateral salpingo-oophorectomy, would she have suffered the same level of depression? I did notice, once the door was closed for her to have children, her depression came crashing down like a mega-tsunami, tossing her into the fight of her life for survival.

I believe she may have had underlying depression, which was blown sky high by the insecurity of being unable to have any more children and loss of hormones from menopause. Her belief that her husband was unhappy with her inability to have any more children, and her feeling that her daughter did not love her, all leading to a perfect storm.

When one suffers in the family, everyone suffers. D.V's husband carried an enormous burden of protecting her from harming herself, and D.V's daughter had to live with the fear she could lose her mother at any time. These were the lives lived in fear, scarred by the experience, but eventually, were able to find healing because of the foundation of love, courage, and faith. It was also the commitment of family members not giving up on each other during their most difficult times.

As her physician—a professional bystander—watching her going through life-and-death challenges made me aware of the complexities of mental illness. D.V's journey of struggles and triumphs over her mental illness was a result of the fighting spirit of D.V and her family during times of deep despair. D.V and her family showed me the real faces of life's survivors and winners.

During my career, I realized it is not just the physical challenges like cancer, cardiovascular conditions, or surgical emergencies that bring us to the doorstep of life or death. Mental illness is made even more challenging with the taboo and secrecy surrounding it, making it more difficult for patients and families to overcome the shame and seek treatment.

D.L's struggle through anorexia or D.V's' struggle through her depression is no less daunting than J.J's struggle and recovery from her accident, not defined by her paraplegia or C.C's son's struggle and recovery from the brain trauma. These are shining examples of human spirit, strength, and grit arising from love, courage, and perseverance.

H.W's Story: Facing an Unimaginable Challenge of Trust in Marriage

No matter which partner seeks the divorce, divorce is one of the most complicated events in one's life. In my experience, most men start the divorce process in a marriage, but some of my patients sought a divorce, too. The reasons for divorce are very diverse: unhappy couples with poor communication; domestic violence; alcohol or drug abuse; betrayal and affairs; or in a few cases, the unknown sexual orientation of the partner. Divorce becomes even more complicated when the children are involved, with each party trying to be the favorite parent. It often includes innuendos blaming the other parent without thinking about the emotional impact, and the burden they are placing on their beloved children. The grief process in some cases of divorce is worse than death, with no resolution for the person who did not initiate the divorce, causing lasting pain and anger. Others find the strength to move on with the lessons learned from the past and seek new paths to lead a peaceful life. A fortunate few find love again that is lasting for the rest of their lives.

H.W had seen me for many years. I saw her through miscarriages and ultimately several successful births at full term. She was delightful and seemed to be very content with her life and her longtime husband, who was the only man that she had ever seriously dated before she was married. I got to meet him during her tribulations of miscarriages and her triumphs of childbirth. They seemed to be a very loving couple in a stable marriage. I continued to see her for many years after her last child was born. Her children were growing up quickly, and one of them was in college.

A few years ago, during one of her visits, H.W talked to me about the events that had transpired during the year before. Her husband revealed that he had been struggling and leading a dual life as a gay man. As one could imagine, her husband's revelation turned her life upside down. Initially, she was confused and questioned herself. How could she not know the man who was her first love, the man she had been married to for more than 20 years, with whom she shared her bed and with whom she had children, was a gay man?

He revealed to her that, he tried to be "straight," fearing being cast as a sinner, but he had known he was gay all his life. He found himself no longer able to cope with this conflict, the conflict of living a lie, a life he tried so hard to make it work. He expressed how much he loved H.W and the children. While he had honestly wanted to make a life with her, he was no longer able to deny his sexuality. He had been suffering from the bouts of depression and was unable to recover, and all this time, H.W had no clue about the cause of her husband's depression.

Learning about her husband's sexual orientation threw her into a life that she had no control over and had never expected. She had to face new realities while going through the emotions of grief, self-doubt, and anger while at the same time trying to understand her husband's journey of pain and suffering. Here, he had been trying to play a different role than what he indeed was, and wanted to be, all his life. It was worse than death. The husband she loved, as she knew him, died the day he revealed the lie of their love and marriage. She struggled with self-doubt about how she had had no clue about who he was and questioned her judgment regarding love and marriage. Her in-laws did not want to accept that their son was a gay man and firmly believed that homosexuality was a choice rather than something established at birth and prayed to God to change his heart.

However, H.W understood and accepted her husband's sexual orientation. Their children, like most children, could accept it better than anyone in the family. Even after going through the divorce, H.W's husband would lean on her for emotional support while she was going through her grieving process of the loss of a husband, their love and marriage, and, perhaps most important, the trust. After much counseling, H.W was able to accept that it had not been her fault for not realizing her husband's sexual identity. Finally, after a few years, she was able to separate from her ex-husband and his life 's journey as a gay man and was able to move on with her own life. The last I heard from her, she had started dating, once again believing in herself.

Even when the events of H.W's life were spinning out of control and thrusting her into an arena into which she had never expected to be, I was amazed to see this devout wife exhibiting such sympathy toward her husband. H.W understood his struggle, and his journey trying to cope with the role he had attempted to fulfill as a husband and ultimately was unable to do. She showed an amazing grace of understanding and ability to forgive him for causing her such great pain, suffering, and grief. By doing so, she set herself free and was able to move forward, accepting him for who he was. Ultimately, by understanding her husband's sexual orientation was not a choice, but possibly more from genetics, she was able to heal and become whole again. H.W's journey of understanding was an inspirational story to me about acceptance and forgiveness.

For parents, the dreams of a "normal" life (parents definition) for their child get shattered with such news of their child being gay or lesbian, the dreams, which began the day he/she was born. Parents facing this new reality, fear what lay ahead for their child in our society. At the same time, they face the challenge of overcoming any shame they feel around the prejudices that they grew up with, and may have cultivated throughout their entire life. They even fear for their child, if they believe that homosexuality is a sin. An intense grieving process of denial, anger, bargaining, depression, and acceptance is a journey which a parent goes through, even if he/she believes the cause of their child's sexual identity is not a choice.

It may take a long time to come to terms with reality, and the process is different for everyone. Some parents are never able to overcome their denial and are unable to understand their children's struggle to accept their sexual orientation before they reveal it to their parents. In the last decade, with significant changes in our society's acceptance, I see that parents are at least more relieved that their children will face less discrimination.

They are more hopeful that their son/daughter will find happiness like every human being wants and deserves. With the better understanding of sexual identity revolving around the environment and master regulators in genes; parents may be able to accept and love their children with the knowledge it is not a choice.

R.R's Story: Dedication to "Rules of Engagement" Resulted in Children's Success

Divorce, no matter for what reason, often has many victims. The spouse, the children, and the extended family are all affected, even more so if the couple were together for many years. The children suffer the most, navigating a divided home and meeting the loyalty tests demanded by each parent. Parents do not always recognize the burdens of abandonment and guilt, and what children have to bear in a two-home situation. It makes it worse and more difficult to manage the children's feelings when parents are involved in relationships or get married again. Some children of divorced parents struggle, whereas others thrive, depending on the cause of the divorce and the commitment of at least one parent to the well-being of the children. I have seen a few mothers who decided to dedicate their lives to bringing up their children at the cost of their happiness, by not getting involved in any romantic relationship. It was a great sacrifice on the part of the mother. I am not suggesting that is the only answer, but it is critical that both parents decide to have a common goal of making sure their children feel loved, rather than engaging in playing games involving one-upmanship.

R.R had been my patient for many years, and I delivered three of her four children. She worked as an administrative assistant to an executive. Her husband became an alcoholic. It was becoming harder for R.R to live under those conditions, and she had threatened to leave him with no response. She is a devout Catholic, so she struggled with the idea of divorce and was not sure how she could raise four children by herself. While she knew her husband's alcoholism would have a negative impact on her children; she also knew the impact divorce would have on her and the children and she was not sure how to go about finding the right path for all of them.

Finally, she found the help through her daughter's school counselor, who came to know what was transpiring at home. The school counselor referred R.R to a family counseling for her and the children, which gave her the courage to divorce her husband. She wanted to devote her life to making sure her children got all the love they deserved and wanted to pass on to them the values which would enable them to become good human beings. She wanted to have flexible hours and make sure she was available for her children, so she decided to quit her well-paying job and become a cleaning lady.

She was uncompromising and made sure her children understood the difference between right and wrong, the value of hard work and self-reliance and, above all, the importance of family. Her sacrifice and dedication paid off. All her children graduated from college, every one of them has a great job, and all of them are in stable marriages, and she is blessed with five grandchildren. All her children and their spouses love her, and she is very actively involved in her children and grandchildren's lives. R.R is still working as a cleaning lady, and I hope her children understand the sacrifices she made to make sure they had better lives while not thinking about her happiness. To listen to her talking about her children and grandchildren with such great pride and joy makes me feel she had no regrets about her decisions in her life.

W.W's Story: My Failure to Understand My Patient's Needs

As physicians, during the moments of a difficult diagnosis, we try to find the delicate balance between providing the facts of the condition and giving hope for the future. As my practice matured, I had many patients that had the challenging diagnosis of cancer, and I thought I had found the right balance of communicating with them, with the facts, possible treatments, and addressing the emotional responses of fear and anxiety, while offering hope for the future. However, there are occasions when I failed in trying to convey the correct message. I was disappointed in myself when I heard that the patient had been upset by the way I communicated with her regarding her diagnosis and treatment.

W.W, who was in her 40s, had seen me for many years for her yearly gynecology exam. A few years ago, during one of her visits, I felt a small lump in her breast. While reassuring her that most likely lump is benign, we discussed the need for further testing with a mammogram and a breast ultrasound. After she had the tests, our radiology department informed me and W.W, the results were normal. Just as I was ready to call W.W to suggest that she still needed to see a surgeon for the evaluation of the palpable lump even though the radiology tests were negative, the radiology department called me to say that they read the earlier report inaccurately. A small mass showed in the breast ultrasound would need a biopsy for further evaluation. I was relieved to see that the standard double-check process worked in catching errors in diagnosis.

I was worried about how the change in the results would influence W.W's state of mind after she had been relieved to know the test reports were negative for any abnormalities. W.W seemed to have received the change in the results and the need for biopsy well and went ahead with the biopsy. The biopsy revealed an invasive carcinoma of the breast, a Grade 1 tumor. I have always struggled with what is the best way to communicate with the patient when a cancer diagnosis is involved. Should I call them to come into the office to discuss the report? This approach created stress and anxiety for my patients who wanted to know the results immediately rather than waiting to schedule a visit that day or the next day (if I am in the OR). Alternatively, do I talk to them on the phone with a family member present to lend support? Unfortunately, I never settled on the correct approach. I am aware of the benefits of a direct in-person consultation, which always contributes to better communication, but I also realize the anxiety created in a patient, who knows something is wrong but must wait to find out what, even if it is a few hours to one day wait.

In W.W's case, I called her later in the evening at home and asked her if her husband was also home to make sure she had the support after she received the diagnosis that I was about to discuss. During my conversation with W.W, I discussed the facts of the cancer diagnosis and revealed that it was a Grade 1 tumor, which was good news, but explained that we would not know the stage of cancer until further evaluation. To get this information, she needed to see a general surgeon for a lumpectomy and sentinel lymph node dissection. I further explained that having a small tumor with the Grade 1 cell type gives us hope that it is most likely an early diagnosis with good prognosis, but the final determination of the stage of cancer would come only after the lumpectomy, and additional testing. As expected, W.W was anxious, as anyone would be, after hearing the diagnosis and had multiple questions. Her husband was on an extension, listening to our conversation. At the end of the discussion, I said that cancer diagnosis is a journey with many emotional ups and downs, lending emotional support and addressing her fear and anxiety. I honestly thought my message to her was very hopeful, pending the definitive diagnosis.

A couple of days after she had seen the breast surgeon, she called my office in anger and talked to a member of my office staff. She explained that the surgeon had told her that she was going to be okay, but that she was upset by the way I had communicated with her. She felt I had led her to believe the cancer was worse than what she ultimately learned from her breast surgeon. That was the first time; I got a call from a patient with cancer upset about my way of communication. I felt terrible, not because she was upset with me, but for what she must have gone through for a couple of days, thinking her prognosis was poor and imagining the emotional impact of her fear and anxiety for which I was responsible.

After my staff relayed her frustration about our conversation to me, I called her back. I wanted to let her know how very sorry I was that she had gone through the fear and anxiety I had inadvertently created from my conversation with her. She expressed that I did not tell her that her tumor prognosis would be good, most likely she did not hear much of what I said, after the initial word cancer. When I talked about the emotional journey dealing with cancer, she thought I said it because she might be dying of cancer. She was also upset I had called her late in the evening. She did say; she appreciated that I had diagnosed the breast cancer in such a very early phase.

In the past, other patients had told me they felt reassured from my conversations under similar circumstances. As a physician, I thought it was my failure not to understand W.W and to determine the proper way of communicating with her. Possibly had I talked to her in person, rather than on the phone, the conversation might have avoided creating unnecessary anxiety because I could have gauged her response by her body language and facial expression and responded accordingly. I was sorry she had to go through this unnecessary anxiety on the top of the shock of learning about her diagnosis of breast cancer. I took my role as a physician seriously and attempted to address all my patients' concerns. Any failure on my part to meet all the patients' concerns made me aware of my human inadequacies, and it is with humility that I accept my responsibility and apologize to all the patients who were disappointed in me and my failure to connect with them.

Z.Z's Story: The Miracle of Life

During my many years of practice, there are some patients whom I cared for but did not see them for follow-up care. It may be because of the changes in their health insurance, or because I was not their primary physician, or possibly because they were not satisfied with my care. There were some cases where I always wondered how some of the children were doing, especially when a baby had complications at birth. It was one of my most exhilarating and uplifting experiences when, out of nowhere, I would hear from a former patient or a family member, who updated me about the wellbeing of one of the patients I thought about for many years.

In the 1990s, a birth took me to the brink of wanting to quit practicing altogether. Z.Z, who was one of my partner's patients, was in very active labor when I arrived for on-call duty in the evening and took over her care. She was in the FBC, planning to have a natural childbirth. During my evaluation, I realized she was completely dilated and had a very thick meconium-stained fluid present as her amniotic membranes ruptured. Meconium-stained fluid could be a sign of stress to the baby. Though most babies so diagnosed do well, such a baby requires close observation with the electronic monitoring and may need additional care at the time of the birth. I discussed these concerns with Z.Z and her husband and the need to transfer her to labor and delivery at the hospital. It appeared hard for them to accept this recommendation from a physician they hardly knew. They were reluctant to be transferred, which would turn their birth plans upside down. It took a few minutes of convincing to make them understand the need for a transfer, but eventually, they agreed.

I placed Z.Z on continuous monitoring, the baby was stable, and I delivered the baby. I took extra precautions in performing deep suctioning of the meconium stained fluid before the baby took his first breath, in order for him to avoid aspirating the fluid into his lungs. In spite of my best efforts, the baby was having difficulty breathing, suggesting meconium aspiration, and subsequently, had to be intubated and placed on a ventilator to maintain optimal oxygenation. We were unable to maintain adequate oxygenation on the mechanical ventilator. The on-call team of a pediatrician, respiratory therapist, and I took turns using a handbag connected to the ventilator to provide enough ventilation to maintain the oxygenation. I was utterly devastated, thinking that somehow, I had not suctioned adequately and to see this baby fighting for his life. Since then, we have learned through research that meconium aspiration happens in utero, not at the time of the birth. However, we did not know that information at the time of Z.Z's delivery. The parents were confused about the outcome on the night of the delivery and did not comprehend the seriousness of the situation, despite us having multiple conversations.

The next morning, a neonatologist evaluated the baby and decided to transfer the baby to the University of Michigan, so he could be placed on an ECMO (Extra Corporeal Membranous Oxygenation, similar to a heart-lung machine) to bypass his lungs to help them heal. Luckily, the University of Michigan was the very hospital which had just invented this machine to be used in newborns. Z.Z's son, B.Z was transferred to the University of Michigan.

For the first few days after B.Z's birth, I was so devastated, I took off a couple of days to contemplate quitting the practice of medicine altogether. After this initial phase of grief, with the support of my husband, I decided not to leave medicine and returned to work. Meanwhile, after a few weeks at the University of Michigan, B.Z was transferred back to our neonatal intensive care unit. I used to go to visit him in his small hospital bassinet and hear his loud wheezing from the bronchopulmonary dysplasia (a chronic inflammatory lung disease caused by prolonged ventilation and meconium aspiration). B.Z was discharged about a couple of months later with an uncertain future ahead of him. Z.Z chose to switch from my partner and came to see me for her second pregnancy. At that time, I learned that B.Z was doing amazingly well, meeting all the developmental milestones. I delivered her second baby with no complications. After a follow-up visit for her second delivery, I did not see Z.Z again and had no information about B.Z

About 20 years later, a gentleman in his late-40s to early-50s walked into my waiting room and told my office staff that he wished to speak to me. Standing with me that morning, he introduced himself as B.Z's father. He said that when he was walking down the hall outside of my office, he had noticed my name on the door and decided to come in and give me the update on B.Z He asked me if I remembered B.Z Of course, I did. He explained that he just wanted to let me know that B.Z was in college and was doing very well. I was ecstatic to know that B.Z was doing so well and thanked him for remembering me and taking the time to give me this good news.

An Obstetrician's Life: Uplifting Stories

In 2015, I was attending a state-sponsored surgical quality collaborative meeting as one of the physician representatives from my hospital. Multiple representatives from different hospitals were meeting to exchange ideas and discuss best practices to improve quality outcomes across Michigan.

At the end of the meeting, a woman approached me and introduced herself. She went on to say that about 28 years ago, I had been on call for one of my partners when she was admitted to the hospital at 29 weeks' gestation with severe pre-eclampsia. She told me that she had been so scared and was very grateful that I had stayed with her in the room the entire time, reassuring her that she was going to be okay. She remembered me sitting in the chair across from her bed, eating potato chips (now, of course, it is forbidden to eat in patient areas) because I would not leave her to eat lunch. Finally, after stabilizing the pre-eclampsia, I decided to deliver her at 29 weeks. Here, this day at the meeting, she thanked me and then opened her wallet to show me the picture of her beautiful daughter, who was going to school at the University of Michigan to become an audiologist. What a pleasure it was to meet her and listen to her talk about her daughter, her eyes filled with pride.

It was not unusual for me to go to an event and run into someone who would tell me that I had delivered them decades earlier. One of these occasions that stands out to me was when my husband and I were attending the Detroit Economic Club fund-raiser on the invitation of our neighbors, Mr. Joe Welch and Mrs. Clare Welch. We were in a long reception line to pick up our name tags. When my turn came, I gave my name to a young lady, who must have been in her mid to late 20s and who was standing across the table. In this crowd, she picked up my nametag and suddenly said, "Stop," to her coworkers. Leaning across the table, she asked me, "Are you Dr. Gavini, the obstetrician, and a gynecologist?"

I replied, "Yes," not knowing where the conversation was going.

She continued, not giving up her inquisition, "Have you been practicing for a long time?"

I smiled, amused at her emphasis on "long."

At this moment I was in a long line of people, all of whom were waiting impatiently for this conversation to be over.

However, curious, too, perhaps, I replied, "Yes."

Then she said I had delivered her and her three siblings.

She added that her mother still talks about me and her birth experiences.

I was astonished that she had recognized my name amidst the sea of nametags at the end of a long line at this event not related to anything medical. I was also very touched that she had taken the time to let me know what an important role I had played in her life.

The most uplifting moments in the life of an obstetrician are when someone who first appears to be a stranger walking toward you and tells you the vital role that you played in her life during her most difficult times. As an obstetrician, I had the most blessed life, knowing I had been a part of so many mothers', babies,' and families' lives. I was even more aware of it when one of them took the time to let me know I had made a difference in their lives. Their gestures of appreciation certainly made a difference in my life.

New Chapter: Understanding of the Medical-Industrial Complex

I would not be able to do justice in trying to describe the medical-industrial complex accurately in one chapter. The delivery of healthcare in our country is very complicated. The special interests and different stakeholders, such as---Pharmaceutical companies, health insurance organizations, government bureaucracies, hospitals, physicians, and patients— all play a significant role in increased healthcare costs. We rank number one in health care costs and 11th in outcomes in the industrialized nations. In spite of this understanding, we refuse to look at our healthcare delivery with a holistic approach.

I was a part of the healthcare system for more than 30 years, not knowing the real cost of healthcare or its actual impact on the quality of care. If we all work together, it may be possible to change the paradigm of quality improvement while reducing the costs and avoiding a healthcare crisis in our country. Even though the Affordable Care Act is the first step in trying to provide meaningful health care to everyone, it is a long way from achieving the goals of improving the quality and reducing the costs. We do not have to go far to find out how to initiate optimal healthcare. Hawaii is one of the few states that has managed to cover most of its citizens with health insurance and reduced the costs with better outcomes by focusing on preventive health care and by regulating their health insurance companies.

To transform the healthcare industry, all stakeholders have to believe in the transparency of costs tied to the quality of care and its outcomes. I look at it the same way as I do with the food industry. We will do better if we know all the facts about the food we are eating including calories, good fats, bad fats, proteins and of course, sugar in all its forms. Though there are some efforts to improve and change, neither industry is ready to evolve in a significant way.

During my long tenure at Providence Hospital, though I served as an associate chairman of the department, the chair of the quality committee and a member of performance excellence committee of the hospital, I must admit I was not very good at dealing with the hypocrisy and the bureaucracy, two qualities that riddle many organizations. As a woman physician with definite opinions, it was harder to fit into the administration, so I decided to get involved in the areas I felt passionate about, like quality, robotic surgery or issues concerning women's health.

In 2008, Providence Hospital built another hospital—Providence Park Hospital—in Novi, Michigan. Many administrative changes happened during this time. Our regional health system had a new dynamic CEO, Dr. Patricia Maryland from Indiana. When she moved to Detroit, many executives who had worked with her in Indiana moved along with her.

In 2009, we got a new president at Providence Park Hospital. Her name was Jean Meyer. She had moved with Dr. Maryland from Indiana. Ms. Jean Meyer was an oncology nurse with a master's degree, who had moved up in the ranks to become the president of our new hospital. The first time I went to see her in her office was to introduce myself and talk about issues on the patient floors in the new hospital. She opened her notebook and wrote down all my complaints. I must say I was impressed because never before had I seen a president of a hospital jotting down notes.

Shortly after that, I realized she was not just one to jot down notes; she followed through. Jean was somebody I felt comfortable talking to about different issues, big or small, and trusted her to follow up. She did so until each issue was resolved. Not once did I ever notice her not responding to any concern. She was quiet in demeanor, but "a tiger" operationally, who would not give up on the project at hand was completed.

Around the same time, one of the female surgeons, Dr. Linda Dubay, became physician director of the surgery at the new hospital. Though I had known her before, we grew closer, and I came to respect her straightforward approach, even when we differed in representing our departments. She was a good leader, and I liked her qualities of honesty, fairness, and follow-through on issues. Over time, we bonded, and I felt I belonged when I was working with women like Jean, our president, and Linda, our physician director of surgery. We shared a similar mindset and goals, a situation that I had been waiting for such a long time.

In 2010, I became the chief of Gynecology and minimally invasive surgery. Jean Meyer asked me to be a "Physician Champion," and I agreed. I realized how complicated patient care had become and how much of it had become unfamiliar to me. The OB-GYN specialty is the only department that admits its patients and follows them through their entire hospitalization. As a Physician Champion, my responsibility was to go to the patient floor assigned to me and lead the morning rounds with nurses, patient care co-coordinators, social workers, and physician assistants. We went through each patient's diagnosis, treatment, and plans for the day.

It was a wakeup call for me when I learned that most patients were admitted under a physician "hospitalist," who was not the patient's primary-care physician. Most of the primary care physicians did not treat their patients when admitted to the hospital. Hospitalists are physicians, who are responsible for patient care during the hospitalization and are expected to deliver the most efficient and optimal care for a patient's acute illness.

I am not sure if the hospitalist program achieved the intended goals of efficiency and better outcomes. This division of care means that once a patient is admitted to the hospital, they experience a chain of consultations, some necessary and some not, with many prolonging the hospital stay. Even patients with surgical conditions were admitted under a hospitalist service, and the care became more complicated than it used to be 20 years ago. As a physician champion, I tried my best to expedite the care that patients deserved, but to go against the health care industrial complex is as difficult as dealing with the military-industrial complex. A patient's history, the real window into the patient's past and present medical conditions, was lost within this division of care between the outpatient physicians (i.e., primary-care physicians) and the inpatient physicians (i.e., the hospitalists). Just after listening to a patient's chief complaint, physicians would start ordering multiple tests and expensive imaging studies, sometimes without ever touching the patient. Tests are often repeated during the hospitalization without evaluating if the repeat test is going to be relevant to the treatment plan when the patient is stable and responding clinically. This type of routine testing, part of the care management plan, is prevalent in all specialties, for both surgical and non-surgical conditions.

When a patient is hospitalized, it is not uncommon to have multiple physicians and specialists, total strangers to the patient, waltzing through, creating more confusion for the patient, who is already confused and concerned about his/her condition. One must ask: Who is responsible for establishing the communication channels between various specialists? Moreover, who is responsible for developing a care plan and documenting it? Who is the captain of the ship coordinating the care between different consultants and the patient? Most often consultants treat patients independent of each other with very little communication with each other.

While everyone recognizes what the problems are, he or she appears to be afraid of addressing the issues, in part because of the fear of offending one side or the other.

Was This Hospitalization Necessary: Story of an Inpatient

I had my own experiences and disappointments with how we sometimes delivered health care. Most of the of time, we are not endangering life, but sometimes care is inefficient and unsafe. One such example involves a woman in her 80s who was sent to the emergency room (ER) by her primary-care physician because of vaginal spotting. After performing multiple tests, the ER physician diagnosed her to have a urinary tract infection and admitted her to the hospital, starting her on intravenous antibiotics. As a gynecologist, I was consulted to evaluate the patient for the vaginal spotting, which was abnormal considering her age. I went to the hospital to assess the patient the very next morning around 10 a.m. I was somewhat surprised to find out she was not in the room and had already been taken down to the radiology department for an ultrasound of her pelvis before I had a chance to examine her. During a review of her electronic medical records, while I was waiting for the patient to return, I found out that she had had a hysterectomy many years ago.

When the patient was brought back from the ultrasound, I realized by talking to her and her husband that the patient had dementia and her husband was the primary caregiver. He was an excellent historian and was up-to-date on all her medical conditions and surgeries. He said his wife saw her primary care physician the day before the admission for vaginal spotting, who advised her to go to the emergency room. The day she was sent to the ER; she had had some spotting after he cleaned her bottom. My examination revealed she had a small abrasion on her vulva, which was no longer bleeding, and the pelvic exam was normal.

Given that she had had a hysterectomy, I knew her vaginal bleeding was not a symptom of cervical or uterine cancer. I reassured them that the spotting was from the abrasion and that she would be okay and did not need any further treatment. Every physician including her primary-care physician, the ER physician, and the admitting physician failed to connect her symptoms to her history. As a result, she was unnecessarily admitted to the hospital, had unnecessary tests, and was treated for an unsubstantiated urinary tract infection with intravenous antibiotics, causing more harm than good. Her hospitalist ordered an ultrasound (even though she had a hysterectomy) before I even had a chance to evaluate the patient.

I had no control over changing her treatment for the urinary tract infection, but I did personally communicate with the admitting physician about the patient's diagnosis, her history of hysterectomy, the unnecessary ultrasound, and the unlikelihood she had an acute urinary tract infection. If the physician only listens to a patient's chief complaint without paying attention to the patient's history, it could lead to unnecessary treatments, while not executing timely necessary treatments.

In 2010, I became involved in a project that was my dream come true. St. John Providence Health's parent health system, Ascension, the largest Catholic health system in the country, started co-management projects, a joint venture between the hospital and groups of physicians to work together to improve the efficiencies of care and impact the outcomes of the patients. For the longest time, despite the symbiotic relationship between physicians and hospitals, they had never seen eye-to-eye, with little understanding of each other's needs or challenges. The two treated each other with suspicion rather than working together as a team.

Dr. Maryland, CEO of our regional (St. John-Providence) health system, decided to start the co-management projects in the hospitals of our local health system. Providence Hospital CEO Dr. Mike Wiemann chose to start a co-management project involving most surgical specialties, excluding orthopedics and neurosurgery. A strategic council of physician leaders of different surgical specialties and the hospital administration was established in June 2010.

As chief of gynecology and minimally invasive surgery, and a member of the OR Council, I was asked to be one of the members of the Strategic Council for Surgical Co-Management. The Strategic Council included physician leaders, administrative leaders, legal counsel, an evaluation firm, and an accounting firm, which met for ten months to develop by-laws for this new joint venture including the eligibility criteria for physician members and the constitution of the board. During the ten months, we established the board structure and the benchmarks for operational and quality projects. Our board included nine physician representatives and three top executives from the administration: CEO, COO, and CFO. Our co-management company officially started on May 1st of 2011. Dr. Gary Goodman, a cardiothoracic surgeon with an MBA, was elected as board chair and Dr. Linda Dubay as medical director. I became one of the nine physician board members.

Every committee involved physicians, administrators, and nursing staff and aimed to improve quality outcomes while reducing costs. Every physician member was encouraged to participate in one or more sub-committees. Our OB-GYN department members were the most engaged and chaired many subcommittees.

I soon became very engaged in the co-management project. I felt the same energy that I had felt when we started the FBC and was excited to be a part of a team committed to making a difference in patient care while reducing the costs. Of the many projects I was involved in, one of the closest to my heart was the hysterectomy project. Dr. Ralph Pearlman, chief of colorectal surgery, who has a very keen mind and possesses a vision that is different from the most physicians, would lead the colorectal surgery project. We were both charged with developing strategies to reduce the length of stay of our patients. Ralph recommended we decipher all the available data for quality and cost, educate physicians with blind individual data with the benchmarks, and make sensible recommendations on how to improve the cost and the quality outcomes. The hospital agreed to give us the data, which was something that never would have happened in the pre-co-management era.

The hysterectomy project was one of the most significant challenges I have ever undertaken. I was computer illiterate, and I knew nothing about Excel spreadsheets. I considered them just "some computer data thing," which I had never actually read, forget about how to use the data to create a spreadsheet. I felt I should be the person to compile the data for the hysterectomy project. After all, this was my department, and I would have a better understanding of what would be the pertinent data for hysterectomy. The hospital sent me information for 2,000 patients with 20 different variables included. It was time for me to learn how to sort and cut the data. I learned the modern way - by watching YouTube videos. From July to the end of September 2011, I successfully worked with different data sets and was ready for my presentation.

I learned from this experience that it is important to challenge oneself by diving into an area with which one is most uncomfortable. The next step in the project was to present the data to a subcommittee comprised of many of my department members. I presented the data to our department chair Robert Welch, and to my department subcommittee members.

Then I outlined our goals: to maintain or improve quality outcomes, to reduce the length of stay, re-admissions, and the cost of care. I discussed the following steps to achieve the goals:

1) Real-time physician education, by distributing blind data to each physician, which would allow them to compare their data

to the best outcomes based on a case mix index comparing "apples to apples."

2)Nurse education, which involves physician-nurse team rounds to ensure consistency and reliability of patient care

3)Patient education, to set expectations for their operative course, discharge, and follow-up by developing a patient educational DVD

In some ways, this approach was no different from our approach at the FBC where the patient-physician-nurse team worked together to achieve optimum goals. It was also very different than the FBC. The FBC involved a committed group of physicians and nurses, as well as patients in a limited setting, concerning one condition: pregnancy. Whereas, co-management involved multiple surgical specialties and physicians, nurses and patients with different backgrounds, goals, and commitments.

My department committee members took up different projects, evaluating the patient charts for quality, readmissions, instrument usage, the cost of care in the operating room and the floors, and compare CMI and DRG based best practices and the worst practices (comparing apples to apples). Then the committee developed recommendations to improve the quality and the cost outcomes for all patients. The committee members did a fabulous job.

In 2011, Jean Meyer, President of Providence Park, recommended me to be a member of a newly forming OB-GYN fourteen-member physician group representing different regions of the country organized through Ascension Health to exchange ideas about how to improve quality and reduce costs. In October 2011, a meeting was led by Ascension Health leadership focusing on quality excellence. It brought all OB-GYN members of the affinity group and ascension health, to meet and greet each other, as well as to discuss goals and expectations. With the approval of the Ascension health administrative team, I presented our benign hysterectomy master data from Providence Hospital. My presentation was well received by the Ascension administration and the physicians who were present at the meeting. It was a great learning experience for me.

Within a month after my presentation at the Ascension health meeting, and subcommittee members I presented the master data to the department along with the subcommittee findings. Subcommittee members reviewed the outcomes of best and worst practices, recommendations, and opportunities for improvement. As part of the physician education, I distributed his/ her blind data to the individual physician, along with the best practice benchmarks of our department, as well as supporting literature.

Dr. Ralph Pearlman, with his unbound energy, presented his colorectal surgery outcomes to his department. Many times, while exchanging ideas in preparation for our presentations, we disagreed without losing respect for each other. I indeed came to consider him as my friend, and it was my privilege to work with him.

To work as a team to develop a care plan, including accurate and timely communication with the patients and with each other seems simple, but it is much more complicated. It is not easy to overcome the challenges of educating the physicians who are resistant to change and the nurses who are too busy and entrenched in their daily routines. Moreover, patients or their families add to the challenge, when they have not invested the necessary time or attention to their health; and possess the belief that new technologies and treatments can cure everything until they do not.

Not everybody bought into the idea, and some of the healthcare team members perceived us as disrupters who were trying to change the system when there was nothing wrong with it. I must admit that I was particularly impatient when physicians were resistant to change despite the evidence presented to them. We continued to believe the best way to bring about the change necessary to achieve our goals was through real-time education using data and literature.

While every healthcare professional and hospital administrator wants to do what is right for the patient, we do fall short of what we could achieve because there are so many different stakeholders, each with different interests. Hospitals are beholden to the specialties and the physicians with high revenues while the physicians of certain specialties exploit their power to influence the hospital and negotiate to their advantage. This symbiotic relationship and interdependency create a structure wherein low revenue specialties or physicians have difficulty finding their voice to have an impact. Since the implementation of the Affordable Care Act with more focus on value-based care than volume-based care, the primary-care physicians increasingly had seats at the table in the hospital administrative arena.

From 2011 to 2016, I held many different positions in surgical co-management: a board member, the Chair of Quality and Operations, and as the Board Chair from 2014 to 2016.

Many physicians, physician leaders, administrative leaders and staff, nursing and quality leaders and staff, too numerous to mention worked countless hours together as a team, passionately believing in our contributions to make a difference in patients outcomes. Their participation in our many co-management projects improving the quality and reducing the costs helped to achieve the many goals we set for ourselves, along with some failures.

It does not mean there were no frustrations along the way. Between naysayers and a disappointing resistance to change, we had some challenges despite all the evidence we presented. Even with some setbacks, the co-management did more to improve quality and continuum of care and to reduce the costs of surgical services. Surgical Co-Management became one of the trusted organization, and it was not uncommon to hear from the different departments that a co-management team "gets things done."

I want to mention, how honored I was to work with the co-management physician leaders: Dr. Gary Goodman, Dr. Kevin Nolan, and Dr.Ralph Pearlman. I also like to thank the primary-care physician leaders: Dr. Cherolee Trembath (Chairman of Family Medicine) and Dr. Vilma Drelichman (Chief of Infectious Diseases) for their contribution. Of course, we could not have done this without the active engagement of the administrative leaders: Dr.Wiemann, Mr. Joe Hurshe, Mr. Doug Winner, Ms. Margaret Klobucar, and Ms. Tammie Steinard. My special thanks to our outreach manager, Mr. Ben Pearlman, and performance excellence leader, Donna Robertson, R.N., for working long hours with commitment and the dedication that was crucial to our successes. I like to extend my appreciation to Andrea parks our administrative assistant for keeping up with all the nuances of running the comanagement and its schedules

I learned that any one of us could challenge ourselves, diving into the very work with which we are most uncomfortable. Computers, data, Excel spreadsheets, each was undoubtedly a challenge to me. By getting involved in studying the patient data, a whole new world opened to me and helped me to understand how data can collectively help us to improve the patient care, the very thing every physician strives to do.

My Journey Toward Retirement and My Mother's Blessings

In the middle of 2015, as I was in my mid-60s, I began to have a nagging thought in the back of my mind. What will be the next step in my life? What awaits me? Retirement is one of the most transformational events for every working man and woman. I have seen people who are sure when they are going to retire and already have plans for their retirement years. Most of them plan to spend time with family or grandchildren, go golfing, or whatever they had dreamed of doing all their lives and had been unable to, due to their work restraints. Other people want to retire but worry about their finances, whether they will have enough to support themselves for the remainder of their lives.

Retirement is a huge decision in a physician's life. We all talk about it, but when it comes right down to it, we are scared to retire. For most of our adult lives, we have worked very long hours under the very most stressful conditions, dealing with life-and-death circumstances, profound human connections, and the benefit of mostly positive feedback from our thankful patients. We are in a noble profession, and it is hard to walk away from a life so well-defined by day-to-day responsibilities, from the minute we get up in the morning to the time we go to bed at night. Patients always come first, often compromising family responsibilities, which results in missing children's activities and feelings of guilt for not keeping the promises made to one's spouse to attend planned events. Physicians, perhaps more than people in many other professions, mostly define themselves by their work; work is their identity, their life. It is not uncommon to question and wonder what awaits oneself after retirement. I had seen some physicians return to work after they had retired because they were bored, and life felt purposeless.

I did not think about the retirement until the year of my retirement. A few years before I retired, patients would ask my staff or me if I was thinking about the retirement and my answer was always "Not yet and when the correct time comes, I hope I will know." My patients used to agree and were happy to know that I would be around for at least another year. It is true that I did not think much about the retirement, but I felt the need to fulfill specific requirements before I retire. As I was in a solo practice, I wanted to make sure there was a physician who would take over my practice to ensure a smooth transition for my patients and to make sure my staff would continue to have jobs.

When physicians retire, I had seen patients go through grief, separation anxiety and depression. They feel very apprehensive about seeing a new physician, with whom they had no relationship, and worse, felt lost when they had to find a physician on their own with no recommendation. I wanted to minimize the effects of such a transition for my patients, though I had no idea how to do it and did not think about it much. I trusted that things would fall into place when the time was right.

Meanwhile, I had been busy, working 14 to 16 hour days, seeing the patients three days a week, performing surgeries, serving as chief of Gynecology, and a leader of Providence Hospital's robotic surgery program. I was also deeply involved as a board chair of the Surgical Co-Management and managing the surgical co-management projects. I was a very hands-on physician, a trait which extended to taking on some critical projects, taking up many hours of my time in the meetings and implementation. In addition to these responsibilities, I was the chair of the Ascension Health's OB-GYN group and a member of the physician counsel for the physician network at our regional health system of six hospitals, the St. John-Providence Health System. My plate was full, but I enjoyed every single aspect of my involvement in our local, regional and national health systems. My firsthand experience in the operating room and on the floors gave me an insight and the understanding of how the processes we envisioned and planned were being implemented and impacted the patient care.

The events that transpired in mid-2015 for the first time gave me an opening into having an option to retire, if and when I decided to do so. In mid-2015, I learned that Dr. Abby Crooks-Babu, a mother of four, had recently left a group practice due to the conflict inherent in her hectic schedule of practicing obstetrics and her responsibilities as a mother. I had known Abby as a resident and worked closely with her when I was the director of the academic clinic for OB-GYN residents. I recognized her as an excellent resident physician although we had not worked together during the intervening years. I decided to reach out to her to see if she would be interested in practicing gynecology only and join my practice. I was hoping she would say yes. If she decided to join us, I felt I would have fulfilled my expectations of having a competent physician in my place to ensure a smooth transition of care for my patients and my staff would still have jobs. After a couple of meetings with the hospital administration and me, she said yes.

Abby started in my office in June of 2015. I was at a crossroad in my professional life. I started wondering what my future would be. I would be completing my obligation as a Chair of the Surgical Co-Management Board on June 30th of 2016. I had been actively engaged in surgical co-management for six-years if I were to include the first year of strategic planning. The experience was intense and was well worth it, but I felt it was time for me to leave the co-management and provide the opportunity for others.

Around the same time, there were some changes in my department too. In January 2015 my department chair for 20 years, Dr.Robert Welch, decided to move on and join another institution. I got to know his wife Sally well and became a friend to me, and four of us (Rob, Sally, me and my husband) socialized once in a while.

I had all these questions about the retirement and what would be the optimal time for me. As a surgeon, I wanted to retire before my technical skills slowed down. Many surgeons semi-retire and continue to see patients in the office and perform minor surgeries. Though this may be a good idea, I wondered if I would be happy, seeing my patients in the office, and having to refer them to other surgeons if they needed surgery. I came to a decision that I would have a hard time being a part-time physician and retiring would suit me better.

In December 2015, my husband and I went to Sarasota, Florida, for a week. We had bought a condo in Sarasota in 2013, so we would be able to spend more time there during the winter months after we retired. During the vacation, I had time to think about my future and talked to my husband about my plans, saying that I wanted to retire. He said he was okay with that plan if that was what I wanted to do. He did express concerns if I would be able to adjust from having such a hectic life to a life of leisure? I was not sure, but, from that week on, I started giving serious thought to my retirement plans. In January of 2016, Jean Meyer, CEO of the Regional St. John-Providence Health System (promoted in 2013), informed me that Dr. Patricia Maryland, President and COO of Ascension Health (promoted in 2012), had asked us to present our surgical co-management data to the National Ascension Health Executives Meeting in Nashville.

On January 28th, Jean Meyer, as CEO, and I, as a board chair, presented our data on behalf of all the surgical co-management physicians, staff, and administration. Although there were few other co-management comanagements in Ascension Health, we were recognized as the best in the system. It was one of the best-received presentations of the day, and afterward, many of the executives enquired how they could emulate what we had achieved. My answer was simple—it all starts with exceptionally passionate, engaged physician leaders working in coordination with the supportive staff, both working in lock-step with the administrative leadership.

I was both proud and humbled by the reception of my presentation and subsequent positive feedback. Co-management could not have achieved the accomplishments that my presentation showcased without the hardworking team of physicians, staff, and administration. Nonetheless, it was nice to be personally recognized by the leadership of the national health system. Coming only after patient care, this was one of the highlights of my professional life. After I returned from Nashville, I finally decided to retire. I felt I could move on, feeling satisfied with my career. I had been faithful to my beliefs, worked with passion, and tried to make a difference.

Some physicians and members of the hospital administration may have misunderstood my passion for making a difference as disruption and my commitment as interference. We all crave affirmation from our colleagues, and, social science has shown, women tend to look for that validation more so than men. I noticed most women in power still look for validation from the men who work with them, but I have never observed where men needed this same type of affirmation from women in the workplace. The workplace represents the society norms where a woman is paid less than a man for doing the same job. I am most thankful to Jean Meyer, our CEO, for giving me the opportunities I had and for giving me a seat at the table.

After my decision to retire, I started the painful task of informing my associate, Dr. Abby Crooks-Babu, and my staff about my pending retirement on June 30th. I told Abby that it gave me great comfort to know that she would be taking over my practice and how my patients felt comfortable knowing she was there. I expressed my gratitude to my dedicated staff who had invested their lives in my practice. I also told my team that it had given me great comfort knowing they would continue to be a part of the transition process, providing the support to my patients with their friendly smiles. I also informed administrative members of the hospital and Dr. Patricia Maryland, COO, and President of Ascension Health, about my decision. I was stunned when I received a personal call from Pat, who expressed disbelief about my pending retirement. Her generosity deeply touched me and overcome by sudden grief; I choked up and was unable to speak, saying very few words. Pat is a phenomenal leader, and even more importantly, a good human being who is very comfortable with herself. She is indeed a leader's leader. I came to understand why so many people had moved with her from Indianapolis to Detroit.

I had first experienced her charm when she invited my husband and me to her house for dinner. I did not know her that well, and my husband Vinay was closer to Pat than I was. I was hesitant to go to their home, but Vinay reassured me that it would be okay and that Pat and Sam are lovely. The minute we walked into their house, she was so warm and friendly and made me forget she was the CEO of the regional health system and the market leader for the entire state of Michigan. Pat and Sam were terrific. Before she became president and COO of Ascension Health, we had a couple of dinner get-togethers with Pat and Sam, and we had a great time. There are very few people whom I have met who have such a personal charm, conversational ease, a friendly smile, and an ability to make other people comfortable. She is a special person, and I respected her, admired her, and considered her a friend. In 2017, Dr. Patricia Maryland, an African-American woman, was promoted to be the CEO of Ascension Health, the largest Catholic health organization in the country.

The hardest part of my journey toward retirement was to inform my patients of my decision. During this stretch, I experienced a rollercoaster of emotions, happy, and sad, laughing and crying at the same time. We were nostalgic and shared the stories about the good old times, our experiences, of childbirth and family events, tragedies, and triumphs. All this reminiscing, the hugs, and the cards made me recognize once again how fortunate I have been in my life.

An Unexpected Encounter

During my good-bye conversation with one of my patients, a most unexpected event happened. V.W had been a patient for many years. She lost her father from the complications of malignant melanoma. Her mother, who had also been my patient, never recovered from her husband's death. Her mother, in profound grief, ignored her health and died from a condition that could have been treated and preventable. After her mother's death, V.W became very depressed and very angry, feeling betrayed by her mother for not seeking care. V.W felt her mother did not love her enough to want to live. It took a few years for V.W to overcome her grief.

The afternoon I informed V.W about my pending retirement, was in the middle of office hours in a day full of appointments. To my surprise, she said she had already known about my plan, but she was waiting for me to announce it. She continued to say that she could connect through a medium with spirits of those who had died. After her mother's death, trying to get some answers, she sought another person's help to connect with her mother through a medium. At that moment, I was not paying much attention to what she was saying. For one, I am a spiritual person, but not being religious, I never entertained any thoughts about an afterlife. I have always believed there is a force beyond our understanding, which I refer to as "God," who oversees this amazing universe. This force (God) manages the universe with perfect synchrony between the planets and the life and death of all that inhabit our world. Consequently, I was somewhat lost when she started talking about the mediums and the spirits. Then she continued to say that, at that very moment, my mother was talking to her and my mother wanted me to know how very proud she was of me. When I understood what she was saying, I was more than a little suspicious, thinking what mother is not proud of her children.

My mother, who died in 2003, does not come into my dreams very often. I remained suspicious until she started describing my mother to a T, including her physical looks, her personality, and events that had happened in her life when she was young. V.W reported my mother was with a small boy. Suddenly I remembered what I had forgotten; my parents had lost a newborn child before I was born. I was in a state of fog with such an incredible and very accurate description of my mother and her experiences! How could I not believe V.W, who is from a different culture and religion, who lived a world apart from my mother, and who never met or knew my mother? V.W said, my mother, a quiet person, which was true, was talking away and wanted me to know how proud she was of me and how hard I worked all my life. She wanted me to know she has my back and it was okay to move on.

So, my mother, my teacher, my guide, and my friend, who loved me unconditionally, was giving me her blessing, just the affirmation that I needed now during this significant transformational time. Even today, I am confused by this event, and it is hard to believe what happened really happened. However, that day, at that moment, I believed in what was transpiring, and I am grateful to V.W for being such a medium of connection. Moreover, I will be forever thankful to have received the blessings from my mother.

A Window Opens

During the final few months of conversations with my patients, they would ask me what my plans were for retirement. My usual reply was, "I do not know, but I shall find out soon." A couple of patients every day would suggest to me that I should write a book, combining my pragmatic approach to medicine with up-to-date care and positive biofeedback. The idea appealed to me, but the challenge was I had never been a writer and such an undertaking would be a more significant challenge as English was my second language. One of my patients, Maureen Dunphy, came to see me for her annual visit. I had known her for about 35 years, and during our conversation about my retirement, I brought up the subject that if I did not have such handicaps writing a book, I would have ventured into such a project. Then she told me that she taught writing classes at the university and in the community and had just published a book about islands in the Great Lakes Basin. She said she could help me in editing, and after she left, I made the decision to take her up on her offer to help. It is so true that when a door closes, a window opens.

The Emotional Rollercoaster of Winding Down

After that episode and my ensuing decision, I gained a newfound strength that I would be able to get through this most challenging period my life. I decided not to perform any major surgeries after mid-May to make sure I complete all my patients' follow-ups. I also decided not to see any patients in the office in the last two weeks, so that any test results would have been followed up and taken care of before my departure. One of our primary care physicians referred D.W., to me for surgery for very symptomatic large uterine fibroid tumors. D.W., a nurse by profession, decided to have a hysterectomy, after discussing all her options. Though I saw her only once as a new patient, we immediately bonded, and she wanted me to perform her robotic hysterectomy. On May 25th, I performed my last major surgery, and there were no complications. It was a strange feeling of emptiness to acknowledge that D.W. was my last patient and that I would never touch these instruments again. However, knowing that I was doing it my way felt right, like the way I had closed the chapter of practicing obstetrics 18 years earlier. I was completing my job with no stones unturned.

The month of June, my last month in practice was difficult. Though I was trying to keep my emotions in check, it was not easy. I told the hospital administration and OR leadership that I preferred not to have any farewell teas or parties and it was my wish to leave quietly. Providence Hospital had been part of my life for 41 years, and now our relationship was coming to a close. I thought of all the friends and mentors who had been part of my life and who had made me the physician and person I am today.

Every year in June, we celebrate the graduation day for our residents, who are moving into a new chapter in their lives, just like I had done myself about 38 years earlier. I attended resident graduation day every year unless I was out of town or sick. This year, I was not sure I would be able to attend because I felt like an emotional disaster. With the encouragement of my partner, Abby, I went to the graduation to celebrate the achievements of the most recent graduating class. During the ceremony, they incorporated a video tribute to me, which was a total surprise. I was deeply touched by the extraordinary efforts taken by one of the attending physicians, Dr. Jennifer Kaplan, who had put together a videocast, a compilation of interviews with current and past residents, my physician colleagues, and nurses. I was dumbfounded. I said a few words, but to this day, I have no recollection of exactly what I said. This experience utterly humbled me. I believe it was less about me than it was about the people who took the time to participate in producing this video, and in caring enough to send their good wishes to me.

During the five months after my decision to retire, while I talked to every patient about my pending retirement, many patients did not have the chance to see me during that time, and those who spoke to my manager expressed their need to say a proper goodbye. My manager, Ann Shamus, who had been with me for 17 years, and who knew my patients well, suggested we hold an open house from noon to 6 p.m. I agreed and set a date for June 27th, three days before my scheduled retirement date. I am thankful to Ann for suggesting to hold the event as it was one of my best experiences.

During the open house, I had close to 100 people who took the time to come and wish me well. Abby was there at my side the entire time, too. I believe my patients felt comfortable to see this smooth transition right in front of their eyes, from old to young, and they seemed to feel reassured by her presence and with her ease in making conversation with them. I felt good to see that interaction between Abby and my patients. Though I was somewhat anxious about how the open house was going to turn out, I felt at home talking to everyone who came. Much to Abby's surprise, I remembered all their names and was able to share the stories of our collective journey together, the births, the cancers, and the celebrations. Those joyful conversations made my heart swell with all the memories of our journey together, and what we learned from each other.

A Woman of Substance

June 28th was my birthday. Sr. Xavier Balance started as the CEO of Providence Hospital in 1975, the same year I had started my residency. We got to know each other well and became friends. During the intervening years, she served in many positions, was one of the architects of creating Ascension Health and the chairman of boards in different health systems across Ascension Health. However, she had always considered Providence Hospital as "her baby." About two years before my retirement, she had symptoms of a stroke, and the tests revealed she had brain melanoma. The surgeries and treatment had slowed her down, but she never gave up and worked until the end. She wanted to come to my open house. Instead, I suggested that we go for lunch the next day, the 28th. On the way back, she thanked me for my help during her first hospitalization and told me she kept the angel I had given her at her bedside. I told her of my admiration for her, as a leader ahead of her time, a woman of substance and vision. Two months after, she passed away, and I think of her often.

Patient Messages

I received hundreds of letters and thank-you notes, but unfortunately, do not have the room to share all of them here. However, I was very grateful to everyone who wrote expressing their thanks and good wishes or offered words of encouragement or a walk through our shared experiences, which I will never forget. I do, however, want to share a couple of letters in verbatim with you, a reminder that we do not know the impact our words have on the others.

Dr. Gavini:
What do you say to someone who has taken care of you for over 30 years and delivered four of your babies? "Thank you" pales. Not only did you care during the pregnancies, but all long until the present day, I have always known you were there if I needed you. When I came to you pregnant with my fifth baby, I was, as usual, feeling sick. I said, "I did not mind having another baby, but I hate being pregnant." You replied, "You do not have to like it, you just have to do it." That was such a blessing to me. It got me through not only that pregnancy but many other tough situations. Such wisdom!

I wish you the best retirement. Know that you have made a difference in my life and so many others. God bless you.

Sandy (Tom too)

Dear Dr. Gavini,

Do you know that I started seeing you well over thirty years ago? Even though for most of these years, I saw you only annually, I have always thought of you as a friend as well as my "special" OB/GYN. Your care and concern for your patients were obvious from my first visit. When you stayed with me in the Birthing Center the night Claire was born, even though you were leaving on vacation the next day, I was astounded and soooo grateful. I know I shared with you that both my father-in-law and my brother are physicians and, of course, I have spent my career working with many physicians. I know how precious time away from work can be for any physician, so your commitment to me (and I am sure all of your patients) was clear. Years later when the mass in my uterus grew rapidly, and I had to have a hysterectomy, you told me, after the fact, that you were worried and prayed for me prior to surgery. You have no idea what that meant to me. I knew I was in the hands of a competent and skilled physician and never worried about the surgery, but knowing you prayed for me made your care of me even more special.

I will miss our chats about healthcare each time I visit [your office], and I will really miss seeing you every year, my friend. You left a legacy of caring. You have a wonderful heart. I hope and pray for you that you enjoy every moment of your life journey as you move to your next adventures.

With much love and affection,

D'Anne.

However, *I* was the fortunate one. Sandy's letter reminded me of how to manage my retirement, that is I do not have to like it, but I just have to do it, and eventually, I will see the light on the other side. D'Anne's letter stated how my words about the prayer made a difference in her life, which is a reminder and a lesson to me that it is not what we do; but, what we say could have a more significant impact.

That last week of my retirement, Jean Meyer, CEO of our regional health system, came to my office and spent about an hour with me. That day I was a "basket case," of emotions. However, I said to Jean, repeating my own words of which I was reminded by Sandy in her letter that "I do not have to like it, but I have to do it" to get to the other side. Jean had been my friend and my mentor in the past decade, helping me get into the administrative arena of health care. Jean's friendship had held me together many times. Her quiet strength, subtle suggestions, thoughtfulness, and caring conversations are something I will never forget and will always be close to my heart.

I will miss working with Dr. Linda Dubay. Besides working very well together in caring for our mutual patients, we had similar goals in approaching most of the quality and cost projects. Over the last few years, we became close friends. I will cherish Linda's support, honest approach, and friendship.

June 30th arrives. Time to close the door of one of the longest and most important chapters of my life. For the last 41 years, I considered Providence Hospital as my home, and now I am leaving the comfort of the home and heading off to an unknown future.

At this time of considerable uncertainty, I am comforted to know that I have a very blessed life and feel assured that I will not be lost. Not with the wind of my mother's blessing on my back, protecting me, and with my shared journeys with my patients and their stories permanently etched in my memory.

Special thanks and Acknowledgements

To Pat Ardinger, who entered my life over 30 years ago, there are not enough words to express what she meant to me. Pat, I want to thank you from the bottom of my heart, for giving me your unconditional love and support beyond what I deserved. Pat, you were, are, and will always be part of my life.

My heartfelt thanks and appreciation to Ann, my office manager, who was by my side for 17 years. I will never forget her phenomenal work ethic, treating patients as friends, with a big smile on her face. I am forever grateful for her unwavering commitment and loyalty to me and my practice, no matter what was going on in her personal life. Ann, I will cherish your friendship and thank you for being part of my life. I want to thank Sarah, my medical assistant, who is mature beyond her years, for coming into our practice and my life at a critical time, who treated our patients with such a calm demeanor and kindness. Thank you for taking on the challenge to work with me and especially for helping me with the electronic medical records. You are a special person and made a big difference in my life. I like to convey my appreciation to Kelly Plannert, for joining our team in the final year of my practice and for treating our patients with respect and professionalism.

There is no adequate word to express my gratitude to my nursing staff over the years. Agnes, Rita, and Kathy, who guided our patients with their clinical expertise, with the highest level of integrity, kindness, and friendship, and who never forgot that the patient is the center of our mission together. I will always remember what we achieved together and the contributions you made to the superior care of our patients. Special thanks to Kathy Sweeney for her friendship spanned over 30 years, for her extraordinary care and support to the patients, while taking on a challenging job of being my nurse manager. Kathy, I can never forget, how you stood by me when my mother died.

My sincerest thanks to Jo Murphy, whom I had known since my residency when she worked as a labor and delivery nurse, and who was always there for me during my entire professional career, either lending a hand in my office when needed or working in the FBC. Jo, thank you for being my friend, you helped me in more ways than you will ever know with your quiet, caring demeanor and subtle encouragement.

I want to thank Diane Allen, Sue Messler, Katie Ranko, Kathy Irwin, Yvette Bush and Amy Thomas who supported my patients, my office with loyalty and dedication over many years.

My sincerest thanks to the FBC staff with whom I bonded and from whom I learned that medicine is not just science. Practicing medicine is, more importantly, about the person, the heart, and the passion for making people's lives better. Our journey together in that endeavor always made me proud. It was an exhilarating experience to be part of that team, and I will always carry those cherished memories in my heart.

I will never forget the support and friendship of the labor and delivery nursing staff, who nurtured me and supported me from residency training all the way into my practice.

Thanks to my husband for his support, and for reading through the first draft of the entire manuscript. His daily encouragement helped me to believe that I could do it. There are not enough words to express my appreciation to my nieces Anita Gavini and Rekha Gavini, for their feedback, patiently going through the manuscript twice. My thanks to my sister-in-law Anu Gavini, for going through my manuscript and helping me to get the manuscript ready for publication. My thanks to friends Jo Murphy, and Mary Lou Longeway for their willingness to read the entire manuscript and for giving me their honest opinion in spite of their busy schedules.

This book would not be complete without the cover designed by Eric Keller, and I appreciated his patience, his advice, and professionalism in working with me.

Last, but not the least, I would like to thank Maureen Dunphy for encouraging me to take on this new adventure, for offering to help, for uplifting me when my spirits were down, and for painstakingly editing every word and every line of mine, twice. Without her, I could not have completed this project of mine.

Index

CPSIA information can be obtained
at www.ICGtesting.com
Printed in the USA
BVHW04*1736110518
515953BV00002B/3/P

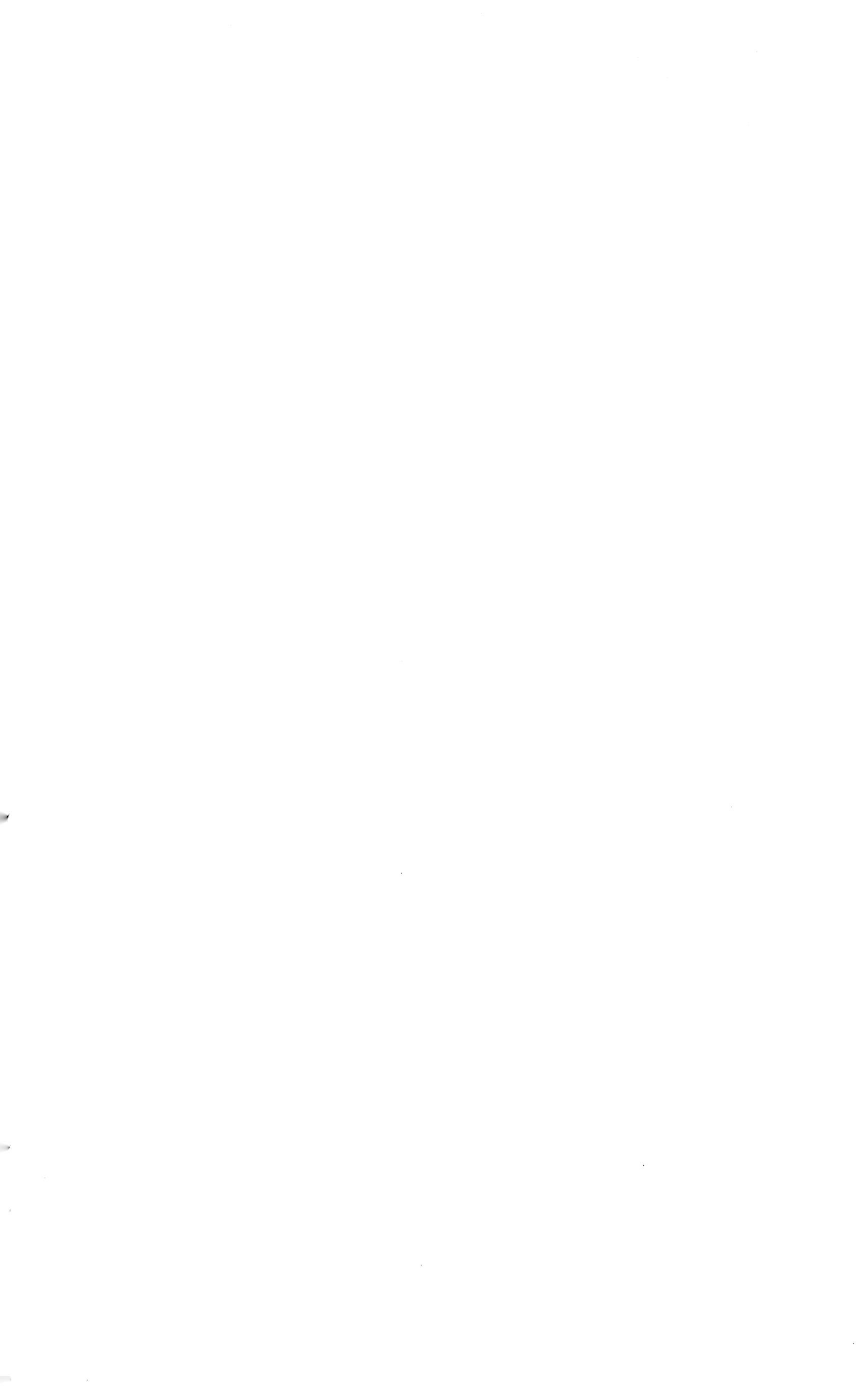